Rapid Review of
ECG Interpretation in Small Animal Practice

Second Edition

T0174408

Rapid Review of
ECG Interpretation in Small Animal Practice

Second Edition

Mark A. Oyama
DVM
Professor
Department of Clinical Sciences and Advanced Medicine
School of Veterinary Medicine
University of Pennsylvania
Philadelphia, Pennsylvania

Marc S. Kraus
DVM
Professor
Department of Clinical Sciences and Advanced Medicine
School of Veterinary Medicine
University of Pennsylvania
Philadelphia, Pennsylvania

Anna R. Gelzer
Dr. med. vet., PhD
Professor
Department of Clinical Sciences and Advanced Medicine
School of Veterinary Medicine
University of Pennsylvania
Philadelphia, Pennsylvania

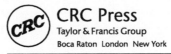

CRC Press
Taylor & Francis Group
Boca Raton London New York

CRC Press is an imprint of the
Taylor & Francis Group, an **informa** business

CRC Press
Taylor & Francis Group
6000 Broken Sound Parkway NW, Suite 300
Boca Raton, FL 33487-2742

© 2020 by Taylor & Francis Group, LLC
CRC Press is an imprint of Taylor & Francis Group, an Informa business

No claim to original U.S. Government works

Printed on acid-free paper

International Standard Book Number-13: 978-0-367-14675-7 (Paperback)
978-0-367-14688-7 (Hardback)

Visit the Taylor & Francis Web site at
http://www.taylorandfrancis.com

and the CRC Press Web site at
http://www.crcpress.com

CONTENTS

PREFACE

Welcome to the second edition, which builds upon the user-friendly format of the first edition and includes new material that will further aid practitioners in their quest to better interpret the electrocardiogram (ECG). This new edition contains additional material regarding acquisition of the ECG, including color figures detailing lead placement and patient positioning. In addition, a handy one-page, two-sided reference guide of important ECG values and diagrams has been included in this edition and can be downloaded from the book's webpage at www.crcpress.com and stored near your ECG machine for easy reference. Several new chapters have been added to this edition. The first covers the basic treatment of arrhythmias, highlighting breed-specific arrhythmias, and includes a table of commonly used antiarrhythmic medications. Another new chapter reviews ambulatory ECG (Holter) monitoring, which can be invaluable in detection and management of intermittently occurring arrhythmias. Practitioners might be surprised to learn that obtaining and placing a Holter recording device on a dog is relatively simple and can be accomplished in most primary practice settings.

Nothing improves ECG skills better than practice, and the core of this book remains, with the extensive series of ECG cases for the reader to work through. For the second edition, 15 new ECG cases have been added to 46 cases already present in the first edition. Some of the new cases call attention to important clinical circumstances involving electrolyte disturbances, supraventricular arrhythmias, accelerated idioventricular rhythms, and atrioventricular dissociation. Another selection of new cases is geared toward readers who craved more advanced topics such as electrical cardioversion and pacemaker function. Even readers relatively new to ECG interpretation will find that exploring these more advanced concepts contributes to better understanding of the fundamentals and will improve their skills. This new edition also includes several cases undergoing ambulatory (Holter) recording and readers will have a chance to consider such data as 24-hour arrhythmia frequency and mean daily heart rates.

This new edition remains true to its roots, our desire to provide information in an appealing, accessible, and easy to use format that fits with the busy lives of veterinary practitioners. To this end, ECGs are reproduced and annotated in full color, and various figures and diagrams are drawn with an emphasis toward rapid interpretation and maximal usability. Finally, we wish to thank the many interns and residents whose cases provided many of the ECG examples we present in the book. Without their work, this book would not be possible.

Mark A. Oyama
Marc S. Kraus
Anna R. Gelzer

AUTHORS

Mark A. Oyama, DVM, MSCE, DACVIM-Cardiology, is a Professor in the Department of Clinical Sciences & Advanced Medicine and Chief of the Section of Cardiology at the University of Pennsylvania School of Veterinary Medicine. He is an Associate Scholar at the Center for Clinical Epidemiology and Biostatistics, Perelman School of Medicine. A Diplomate of the American College of Veterinary Internal Medicine, Specialty of Cardiology, Oyama's clinical specialties involve clinical examinations, echocardiograms, ECG, and noninvasive surgeries. His research spans animal models of heart disease, myxomatous mitral valve disease, cardiac biomarkers, clinical trials, epidemiology, biostatistics, and diuretic resistance.

Marc S. Kraus, DVM, DACVIM-Cardiology/Internal Medicine, ECVIM-Cardiology, is a Professor of Clinical Cardiology and Outpatient Medical Director at Ryan Hospital, University of Pennsylvania School of Veterinary Medicine. He is a Diplomate of the American College of Veterinary Internal Medicine (Internal Medicine, Cardiology) and a Diplomate of the European College of Veterinary Medicine (Companion Animals). His clinical specialties are companion animal cardiology, cardiac biomarkers in small and large animals, and heart failure management. Kraus's research areas include companion animal cardiology, cardiac biomarkers, and antiarrhythmic therapies.

Anna R. Gelzer, Dr.med.vet, PhD, DACVIM-Cardiology, ECVIM-Cardiology, is a Professor of Cardiology at the University of Pennsylvania School of Veterinary Medicine. She is a Diplomate of the European College of Veterinary Internal Medicine—Companion Animals (Cardiology) and of the American College of Veterinary Internal Medicine (Cardiology). Gelzer's clinical specialty is companion animal cardiology, and her research areas include arrhythmias and electrophysiology.

ABBREVIATIONS

AC	alternating current
AF	atrial fibrillation
AFL	atrial flutter
AP	accessory pathway
ARVC	arrhythmogenic right ventricular cardiomyopathy
ATP	adenosine triphosphate
AV	atrioventricular
AVRT	atrioventricular re-entrant tachycardia
BB	beta-blocker
CCB	calcium-channel blocker
CHF	congestive heart failure
CRI	continuous rate infusion
cTnI	cardiac troponin
DCM	dilated cardiomyopathy
ECG	electrocardiography/electrocardiogram
FAT	focal atrial tachycardia
HR	heart rate
ICU	Intensive Care Unit
LAFB	left anterior fascicular block
LBBB	left bundle branch block
MEA	mean electrical axis
RBBB	right bundle branch block
SA	sinoatrial
SB	sinus bradycardia
SSS	sick sinus syndrome
SVA	supraventricular arrhythmia
SVT	supraventricular tachycardia
VA	ventricular arrhythmias
VF	ventricular fibrillation
VPC	ventricular premature contraction
VT	ventricular tachycardia

PRINCIPLES OF ELECTROCARDIOGRAPHY

The electrocardiogram (ECG) is a graphical record of electric potentials generated by the heart muscle during each cardiac cycle. These potentials are detected on the surface of the body using electrodes attached to the limbs and chest wall, and are then amplified by the electrocardiograph machine and displayed on special graph paper in voltage and time. The ECG serves to characterize arrhythmias and conduction disturbances.

INDICATIONS FOR ECG RECORDINGS

- Evaluating arrhythmias and heart rate disturbances detected on auscultation.
- History of syncope (fainting) or episodic weakness.
- Cardiac monitoring during anesthesia.
- Cardiac monitoring in critically ill patients.
- Monitoring changes in rate and rhythm due to drug administration.
- Assessing changes in ECG morphology and heart rate due to electrolyte imbalances associated with extracardiac disease or drug toxicities.
- In addition, the ECG may also be helpful to identify anatomical changes due to myocardial hypertrophy or dilation, and detect pericardial disease. However, echocardiography has largely replaced the ECG for these indications due to its superior sensitivity.

ECG LEAD TERMINOLOGY

In order to record an ECG waveform, a differential recording is made between two electrodes, placed on different points on the body. One of the electrodes is labeled positive, and the other negative. The positions of the electrodes on the body are standardized (Fig. 1.1) and defined as RA = right arm, LA = left arm, and LL = left leg. The output from each electrode pair (differential recording) is referred to as a *lead* and numbered with the Roman numerals I, II, and III. These leads are called limb leads.

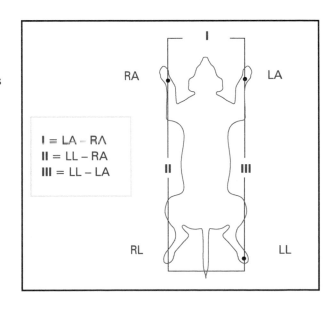

Fig. 1.1 The standardized positions of the electrodes on the body are defined as RA = right arm, LA = left arm, and LL = left leg. The output from each electrode pair is referred to as a lead and numbered with the Roman numerals I, II, and III.

The limb leads form the points of what is known as Einthoven's triangle (**Fig. 1.2**). The positive pole for lead I is on the left arm, the positive pole for lead II on the left leg and the positive pole for lead III is on the left leg. An imaginary line connecting the two electrodes is the lead axis. Each lead looks at the heart from a different angle within the animal's frontal plane. There are 12 standard ECG leads used in veterinary medicine, which provide information regarding the magnitude of the electrical activity of the heart and the direction of a moving depolarization wavefront in multiple orientations. A wavefront traveling toward the positive terminal of a lead results in a positive deflection of the ECG in that lead. When a wavefront travels away from the positive electrode, a negative deflection occurs. A lead axis in parallel to the direction a wavefront is moving results in a large deflection, while a lead axis perpendicular to the direction of a moving wavefront results in a small (or no) deflection on the ECG.

THE LIMB LEADS

There are six limb leads which assess the cardiac depolarization in the frontal plane. A modified version of the frontal plane in the dog is shown in **Figure 1.3**. Leads I, II, and III directly record the electrical activity between two limb electrodes (*Table 1.1*) and are thus referred to as bipolar limb leads. The unipolar (augmented) limb leads use the same electrodes as lead I, II, and III, and also measure the electrical activity between two terminals, but the recording electrode is always positive and the negative terminal is made up of the sum of the electrodes attached to the right arm, left arm, and left leg (**Fig. 1.4**). These limb leads are named after their positive electrode, located on the left arm (aVL), the right arm (aVR), and the left foot (aVF), where the "a" stands for augmented, and "V" stands for vector (**Fig. 1.5**). Together with leads I, II, and III, augmented limb leads aVR, aVL, and aVF form the basis of the *hexaxial reference system*, which is used to calculate the heart's electrical axis in the *frontal plane*. The positive and negative terminals of the six limb leads are listed in Table 1.1.

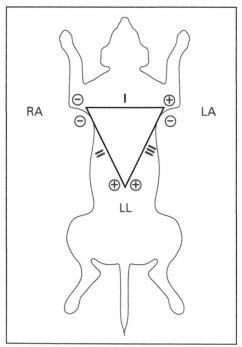

Fig. 1.2 The limb leads (I, II, III) form the Einthoven triangle.

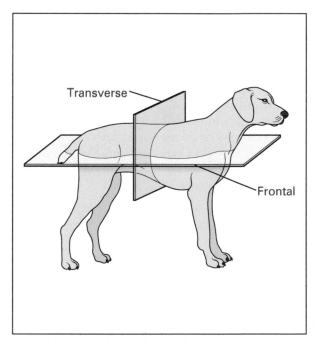

Fig. 1.3 The limb leads display the cardiac depolarization in the frontal plane. The chest leads display the depolarization in the transverse plane.

Table 1.1 The positive and negative terminals of the six ECG limb leads

Bipolar limb leads		Augmented unipolar limb leads	
I	R arm (–) to L arm (+)	aVR	R arm (+) to common terminal (–)
II	R arm (–) to L foot (+)	aVL	L arm (+) to common terminal (–)
III	L arm (–) to L foot (+)	aVF	L foot (+) to common terminal (–)

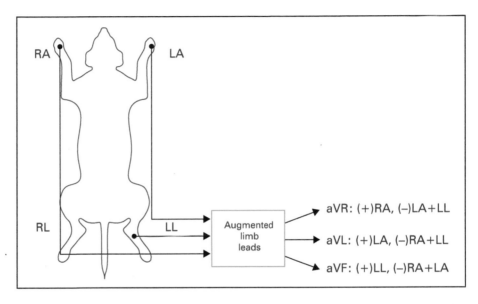

Fig. 1.4 The augmented (unipolar) limb leads use the same electrodes as leads I, II, III, but the recording electrode is always positive and the negative terminal is made up of the sum of the electrodes attached to the right arm, left arm, and left leg.

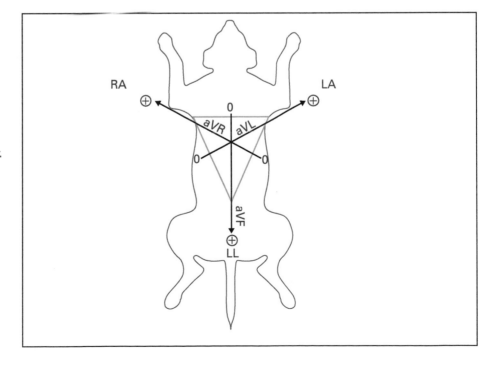

Fig. 1.5 The augmented limb leads are named after their positive electrode, located on the left arm (aVL), the right arm (aVR), and the left foot (aVF), where the "a" stands for augmented, and "V" stands for vector.

THE PRECORDIAL OR CHEST LEADS (V LEADS)

The chest leads view the heart's electrical activity in the transverse plane (see Fig. 1.3, p. 2). This complements the information regarding the electrical fields gained from the six limb leads. The chest leads are termed V (*voltage*) leads. They are considered to be unipolar with the positive exploring electrode placed on the chest (precordium). The electrodes for the chest leads (V1, V2, V3, V4, V5, and V6) are placed directly on the chest (**Fig. 1.6**). In dogs, V1 is placed to the right of the sternum at the 5th intercostal space (ICS). The 6th ICS is used for all the left sided leads V2-V6. V2 is placed just to the left of the sternum, V4 is placed at the costochondral junction; V3 is placed midway between V2 and V4; V5 is placed at a distance above V4 equidistant between V3 and V4; V6 is placed at a distance above V5 equidistant between V3 and V4. Left sided chest leads may be more sensitive than the limb leads for detection of right ventricular enlargement or allow better identification of P waves.

GENESIS OF THE NORMAL ECG

The ECG waveforms are generated by the spread of activation of cardiac action potentials through the specialized electrical conduction system of the heart, as well as the atrial and ventricular myocytes. The specialized conduction system consists of the sinus node, internodal tracts, the atrioventricular (AV) node, the bundle of His, which divides into the two main bundle branches, and the Purkinje fibers (**Fig. 1.7**). Organized electrical activity passing along this specialized conduction system results in coordinated mechanical contraction during each cardiac cycle. The sinoatrial (SA) and AV node cells have the intrinsic ability to fire spontaneously (automaticity). Normal atrial or ventricular myocytes do not spontaneously depolarize. The SA node normally dictates the heart rate because the SA nodal cells have a faster rate of spontaneous depolarization than the AV nodal or Purkinje fibers.

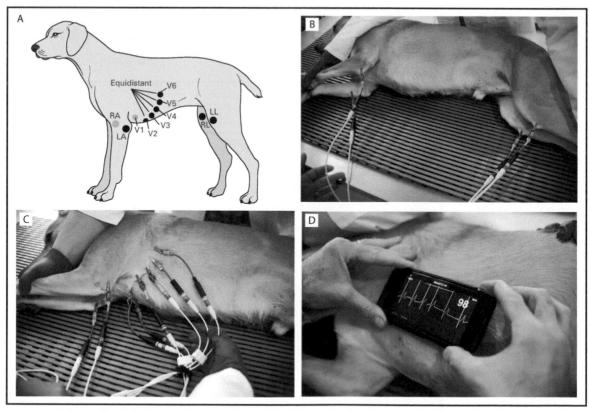

Fig. 1.6 (A) Schematic of limb and chest lead position. The unipolar chest leads (V = voltage) are placed directly on the chest (precordium). (B) Photograph of limb lead placement on a dog in right lateral recumbency. (C) Photograph of chest lead placement. (D) Photograph of a handheld smartphone-based ECG device along the chest wall of a dog.

The actual action potential generated by the SA nodal cells (pacemaker potentials) are too small to be seen on the surface ECG. However, as the activation wavefront encounters the mass of atrial myocardium, the initiation of electrical activity is observed on the body surface. Thus, the first ECG wave of the cardiac cycle is called the P wave and represents activation of the atria. Atrial repolarization is rarely appreciated on the ECG, as it occurs simultaneously with ventricular depolarization and is thus hidden in the QRS complex.

Conduction of the cardiac impulse proceeds from the SA node through the atria via the specialized conduction system of the internodal tracts to the AV node. When the activation wave reaches the AV node, conductions slows markedly, due to the slow depolarization characteristics of the AV nodal cells. This provides time between the mechanical contraction of the atria and the ventricles. On the surface ECG, this conduction delay produces a short, relatively isoelectric segment following the P wave, contributing to the PR interval. When the electrical impulse emerges from the AV node and enters the His–Purkinje network, conduction velocity dramatically increases once again. The bundle of His divides into the right and left bundle branches that depolarize the right and left ventricles, respectively. The left branch further divides into the anterior and posterior fascicule. Once the large muscle mass of the ventricles is excited, a large deflection is seen on the body surface, called the QRS complex. This large wave can have several components. In lead II, there may be an initial downward deflection, called the Q wave, followed by a dominant upward deflection called the R wave. There may also be a terminal downward deflection, called the S wave. The polarity and actual presence of these three components depend on the lead examined.

Following the QRS complex is another short, relatively isoelectric segment, the ST segment. During this time period, the ventricles are absolutely refractory, that is, cannot respond to another electrical activation. After this short segment, the ventricles return to their electrical resting state, and a wave of repolarization is seen as a low-frequency signal, the T wave. During the T wave, the ventricles are only relatively refractory, and may be stimulated by a premature electrical activation. The duration of time from the start of the QRS complex to the end of the T wave is the QT interval which represents the entire ventricular depolarization and repolarization.

Fig. 1.7 The specialized cardiac conduction system.

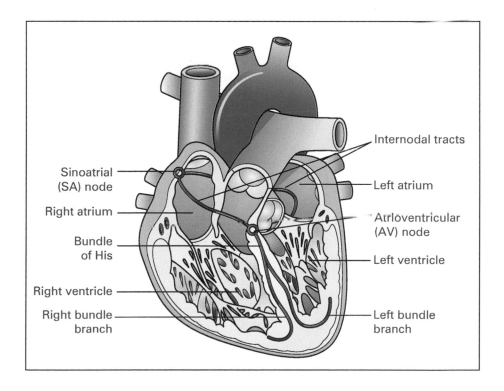

Sinoatrial (SA) node

Right atrium

Bundle of His

Right ventricle

Right bundle branch

Internodal tracts

Left atrium

Atrioventricular (AV) node

Left ventricle

Left bundle branch

LEAD PLACEMENT AND ACQUISITION OF THE ECG

The standard ECG recording systems record an analog signal and use a heated stylus which records on light-sensitive graph paper. Older-style ECG machines recorded one lead at a time while more recent digital systems, which record the ECG on a computer, allow any combination of simultaneous 6- or 12-lead recordings. The ECG machine typically applies a filter to reduce baseline artifact. A 50 Hz filter may be adequate in dogs, but in cats it is best to use a 150 Hz filter in order to include high-frequency components of the R and S wave. Proper grounding is important to avoid electrical interference from 60 Hz alternating current (AC) originating from the electrical supply or other electrical equipment in the room. The ECG reference ground is provided through a separate electrode, either incorporated into one of the three limb leads, or as a separate wire.

Acquisition of the 6-lead ECG:

- Place patient in right lateral recumbency. The animal should have its head and neck resting on a table or on the floor.
- The forelegs and hindlimbs should be parallel and at right angles (perpendicular) to the body.
- The patient must remain still with minimal panting and moving. Cats should not be purring.
- Connect standard limb leads. See *Table 1.2*, Fig. 1.6.
  - Forelimb electrodes at or just below elbows
  - Hindlimb electrodes at or just above stifles

- Once the leads are hooked up properly, the ECG leads should not be touching or crossing over each other.
- If using ECG clips, it is best to wet the skin and ECG clip with isopropyl alcohol or a coupling gel that contains a high ionic concentration to help aid in the transfer of current at the tissue–electrode interface. If using an "ECG patch" these often contain gel within the patch and alcohol is not required.
- Table 1.1 describes the positive and negative terminals that form the bipolar and augmented lead system.

Acquisition of the 12-lead ECG:

- Position patient and connect standard limb leads as described for 6-lead ECG then attach the chest leads as follows (Fig. 1.6):
  - Identify the left 6th intercostal space ($IC6_L$)
  - Connect V2 just to the left of the sternum at $IC6_L$
  - Connect V4 at the costochondral junction of $IC6_L$
  - Connect V3 midway between V2 and V4 at $IC6_L$
  - Connect V5 at $IC6_L$ at a distance above V4 equal to the distance between V2–V3 or V3–V4
  - Connect V6 at $IC6_L$ at a distance above V5 equal to the distance between V2–V3, V3–V4 or V4–V5
  - Connect V1 just to the right of the sternum at right 5th intercostal space ($IC5_R$)

Table 1.2 Electrode position for ECG recording in dogs and cats

ECG electrode	Position
Black	Left front leg at elbow
White	Right front leg at elbow
Red	Left back leg at stifle
Green	Right back leg at stifle

- The left precordial leads should be equidistant along $IC6_L$ with V4 at the costochondral junction, and V2 just to the left of the sternum (Fig. 1.6).
- While the use of alcohol or coupling gel is needed, if excessive amounts are utilized, if the alcohol from one lead comes in contact with another lead, it creates a "lead smear" whereby the QRS morphology from all the leads will look the same.

Acquisition of a smartphone-based ECG:

- Smartphone-based devices that record the ECG from veterinary patients are available (Veterinary AliveECG™) from Apple and Android app stores. A specially designed phone cover or small electrode-containing strip of plastic is placed on the animal's chest. The electrodes relay the surface potential to the smartphone, which then displays an ECG tracing on the phone's screen.
- The phone or electrode strip is positioned over the point of maximal intensity of the cardiac beat on the left thorax with the negative electrode (microphone end of smartphone) placed craniodorsally, while the positive electrode (listening end of smartphone is placed caudoventrally and the phone is angled at approximately a 45° angle (Fig. 1.6). This position simulates lead III. Gentle pressure is applied to insure the electrodes achieve optimal contact with the skin contact. The device position can be readjusted in order to acquire the largest amplitude ECG.

Besides the standard 6- or 12-lead ECG, there are several other uses of ECG recording technology that rely on only a few leads. Continuous monitoring under anesthesia or in the Intensive Care Unit (ICU) using an integrated physiorecording system for blood pressure, oxygen saturation, and so on, typically record only one lead. The ambulatory or Holter ECG is an important technology for long-term monitoring of patients allowing detection and quantification of intermittent arrhythmias. Holters record a two or three lead ECG digitally for up to 7 days. The data can then be stored and analyzed on-line with personal computer-based programs.

The cardiac conduction system and components of the P–QRS–T complex

Through a complex change of ionic concentrations across the cell membrane, an extracellular potential field is established which then excites neighboring cells, and a cell-to-cell propagation of electrical events occurs. Because the body acts as a purely resistive medium, these potential fields extend to the body surface. The character of the body surface waves as seen on the ECG depends on the amount of tissue activated at one time and the relative speed and direction of the activation wavefront. The 12 ECG leads provide information about the magnitude of the electrical activity of the heart and the direction of the moving depolarization wavefront in multiple orientations. A wavefront traveling toward the positive terminal of a lead results in a positive deflection of the ECG in that lead. When a wavefront travels away from the positive electrode, a negative deflection occurs. A lead axis in parallel to the direction a wavefront is moving results in a large deflection, while a lead axis perpendicular to the direction of a moving wavefront results in a small (or no) deflection on the ECG.

An early pioneer of the ECG, Einthoven chose the letters of the alphabet "PQRST" to avoid conflict with other physiological waves being studied at about the same time. The wavefront initiated by the sinus node, located at the junction of the cranial vena cava and the right atrium, depolarizes the atria from right to left and cranial to caudal. This results in a small, upright P wave in the caudal leads I, II, III, and aVF, while it appears as a negative or isoelectric deflection in aVR and aVL. The P wave amplitude is most prominent in lead II, because the average vector of the atrial depolarization is traveling toward the positive terminal of lead II, while the P is almost invisible in leads which are oriented perpendicular to lead II (aVL). While the impulse conducts slowly through the AV node and enters the bundle of His and spreads down into the bundle branches and to the Purkinje fibers, the ECG displays an isoelectric (baseline) line in all leads. These conduction tissues are "insulated" so that the action potential travels mostly intracellular and does not spread into the muscle as a measureable signal on the surface ECG.

Once the impulse reaches the ventricular myocardium, it spreads into the interventricular septum and then across both ventricles, producing the QRS complex on the surface ECG. The initial vector of depolarization into the septum can point cranially and to the right, that is, away from the positive pole of lead II, producing the small negative deflection of the Q wave. Because the muscle mass of the left ventricle exceeds that of the right ventricle, the summation of all vectors of ventricular depolarization point toward the left side and caudally, that is, the positive terminal of lead II, resulting in the large, positive deflection of the R wave. Lead II typically shows the largest R wave amplitude, but normally all caudal leads (I, II, III, and aVF) will depict a positive R wave. The final phase of ventricular depolarization includes the heart base, such that the sum of the vectors is pointed again cranially, producing a small negative deflection, the S wave. Not all dogs and cats display Q waves or S waves as the presence of these waves depends somewhat on the horizontal position of the heart in the chest.

Ventricular repolarization does not occur in the inverse direction as the depolarization, but is a slow process that starts at the epicardium and the ventricular apex, and ends at the endocardium and heart base. The resulting various vectors of repolarization nearly cancel each other out, thus generating the low amplitude T wave in lead II. It can be a positive or negative deflection in dogs, or nearly isoelectric in cats.

Electrical properties of the heart

Two types of action potentials are observed in the heart: The fast response action potential occurs in the normal atrial and ventricular myocardium and in the Purkinje fibers (**Fig. 1.8A**), while the slow response action potential (**Fig. 1.8B**) is found in the SA node, the pacemaker region of the heart, and in the AV node, the specialized tissue that conducts the cardiac impulse from atria to the ventricles (see Fig. 1.7, p. 5).

The various phases of the action potential (Fig. 1.8) are associated with changes in the permeability of the cell membrane, mainly to positively charged sodium (Na^+), potassium (K^+), and calcium (Ca^{2+}) ions. This is accomplished by opening and closing of voltage-dependent ion channels in the cell membrane, selective for individual ions. At rest (phase 4), the Purkinje fiber cells (Fig. 1.8A) maintain an electrical gradient across the cell membranes (*resting membrane potential*) such that the inside is negative with respect to the outside of the cells. This negative intracellular potential is maintained by Na^+ channels, which extrude Na^+ ions from the cell. When an action potential from a neighboring cell arrives, it reduces the resting potential to a threshold (i.e., makes it less negative) resulting in an abrupt increase in permeability of the Na^+ channels, allowing Na^+ ions to rush into the cell and depolarize it. The rapid depolarization (upstroke of *fast response* action potential), that ensues once the cell reaches a voltage threshold corresponds to phase 0. The membrane potential is thus reversed or positive. Once a cell is depolarized, it cannot be depolarized again, until the ionic fluxes that occur during depolarization are reversed, a process called repolarization. The repolarization of the cardiac cells roughly corresponds to phases 1 through 3 of the action potential. Phase 1 consists of a brief rapid repolarization, initiated at the end of the action potential upstroke, as the Na^+ channels inactivate and the K^+ channels transiently allow an outward current. Phase 1 is interrupted when the cell reaches the "plateau phase" or phase 2, maintained by a slow Ca^{2+} influx. The transmembrane current of Ca^{2+} initiates the mechanical contraction of the heart. During the plateau, repolarization slowly progresses, until the Ca^{2+} channels are turned off, and eventually a final rapid repolarization (phase 3) ensues, via an outward K^+ current. Because a second depolarization cannot happen until repolarization occurs, the time from the end of phase 0 to late in phase 3 is called the refractory period. Phase 4 is the resting membrane potential. This is the period that the cell remains in until it is stimulated again by an external electrical stimulus (typically an action potential from an adjacent cell).

Cells from the SA node and the AV node (Fig. 1.8B) have a lower resting membrane potential which becomes gradually more positive during diastole (phase 4) because of steady influx of calcium through slow Ca^{2+} channels, eventually resulting in spontaneous depolarization. The slow influx of Ca^{2+} produces the slow upstroke velocity (*slow response* action potential) in the SA and AV nodal cells.

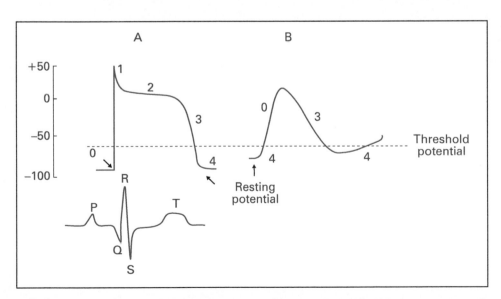

Fig. 1.8 Action potentials of the heart and generation of the surface ECG. The fast response action potential (graph A) occurs in the normal atrial and ventricular myocardium and in the Purkinje fibers and is largely responsible for the generation of the ECG recorded from the body surface. The slow response action potential (graph B) is found in the sinoatrial and atrioventricular nodes.

Section 2

EVALUATION OF THE ELECTROCARDIOGRAM

Evaluation of the ECG is best performed using a systematic approach so that important characteristics are not overlooked. Important features that require analysis include heart rate, rhythm, mean electrical axis (MEA), waveform morphology, and criteria for heart enlargement. This section provides a step-by-step guide on how to evaluate each of these features, but first, one must understand how paper speed and sensitivity settings affect ECG interpretation.

ECG PAPER, SENSITIVITY, AND SPEED OF RECORDING

ECG paper has a background pattern of 1 mm squares and bold division lines every 5 mm in both horizontal and vertical directions (large squares). The ECG is typically recorded at one of two different paper speeds, either 25 mm/s or 50 mm/s. Paper speed denotes the speed at which the paper moves through the ECG machine while the waveforms are being recorded. At 25 mm/s, each 1 mm square represents 0.04 seconds and each 5 mm square represents 0.2 seconds, while at 50 mm/s, each 1 mm square represents 0.02 seconds and each 5 mm square represents 0.1 seconds (**Fig. 2.1**).

ECG sensitivity refers to the amplitude of the waveforms based on electrical voltage. At standard sensitivity, an impulse of 1 millivolt (mV) will inscribe a waveform amplitude that is 10 mm tall (Fig. 2.1). In cases where the ECG voltages are low (i.e., in cats), sensitivity can be increased (doubled) so that an impulse of 0.5 mV will create a waveform of 10 mm amplitude, thereby allowing easier inspection of the individual ECG waveforms. Conversely, in animals with severe heart enlargement, sensitivity can be decreased (halved) so that waveforms do not extend past the borders of the recording paper. Once the paper speed and sensitivity are noted, calculation of heart rate and waveform morphology becomes as simple as determining time and amplitude in number of squares and performing a few easy calculations to convert each value to either seconds or millivolts, respectively.

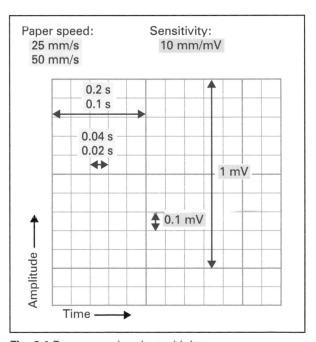

Fig. 2.1 Paper speed and sensitivity.

HEART RATE

If the heart rhythm is regular, the simplest method to calculate heart rate is to count the number of 1 mm squares between two heartbeats (RR interval) and divide this number into 3000 if the paper speed is 50 mm/s (3000 is the equivalent of 1 minute because 60 seconds × 50 = 3000), or into 1500 if the paper speed is 25 mm/s (**Fig. 2.2**). This calculation will yield the heart rate as beats per minute (bpm). If the heart rhythm is irregular, calculation of the average heart rate over a prescribed period of time is performed. It is useful to realize that 30 larger squares or 150 mm represent 3 seconds at 50 mm/s or 6 seconds at 25 mm/s. Thus heart rate is determined by counting the number of QRS complexes over 30 large squares and multiplying this number by 20 if the paper speed is 50 mm/s, or multiplying by 10 if the paper speed is 25 mm/s (**Fig. 2.3**). A commonly used shortcut takes advantage of the fact that many standard ballpoint pens are 150 mm in length. Thus, the pen can be placed on the ECG paper to denote a 3- or 6-second interval and the number of beats that are demarcated by the length of the pen can be quickly counted. To get "bpm," this number is multiplied by 20 if the paper speed is 50 mm/s or by 10 if the paper speed is 25 mm/s.

RHYTHM

The heart rhythm describes the pattern of heartbeats and sequence of the P–QRS–T wave forms. The heart rhythm is best evaluated over a prolonged recording of a 6-lead ECG tracing. When determining the heart rhythm, the following characteristics should be examined:

- The regularity of the heartbeats: Are the RR intervals regular or irregular?
- The relationship of the P wave and QRS complexes:
  - Is there a P wave in front of every QRS complex?
  - Is there a QRS complex following every P wave?
- The origin of the heartbeats:
  – Sinus node
  – Ectopic focus (i.e., atrial, junctional, or ventricular origin)
- The heart rate

In some instances, the heart rhythm changes or is composed of multiple different rhythms that each requires a separate description.

MEAN ELECTRICAL AXIS

The mean electrical axis (MEA) describes the net direction of ventricular cardiac depolarization across the animal's frontal plane (the plane delineated by the four extended limbs if the animal is viewed as lying on its back). The conventional 6-lead ECG system divides the frontal plane into 12 segments, similar to the slices of a pie (**Fig. 2.4**, see Fig. 1.3 p. 2). By doing so, the 6-lead ECG examination records the electrical activity of the heart from six different vantage points along the frontal plane in 30-degree increments (Fig. 2.4). The MEA normally points toward the caudal half of the animal. In the dog, the normal MEA is between +40 and +100 degrees

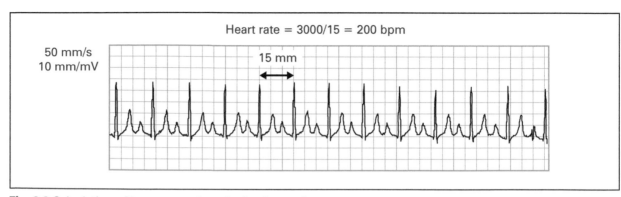

Fig. 2.2 Calculation of heart rate when rhythm is regular.

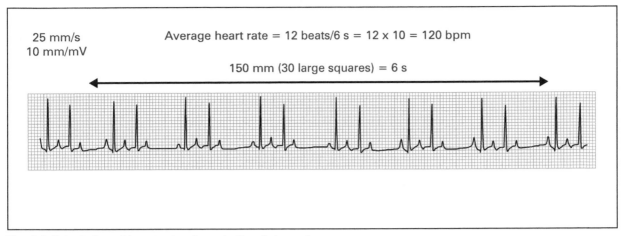

Fig. 2.3 Calculation of heart rate when rhythm is irregular.

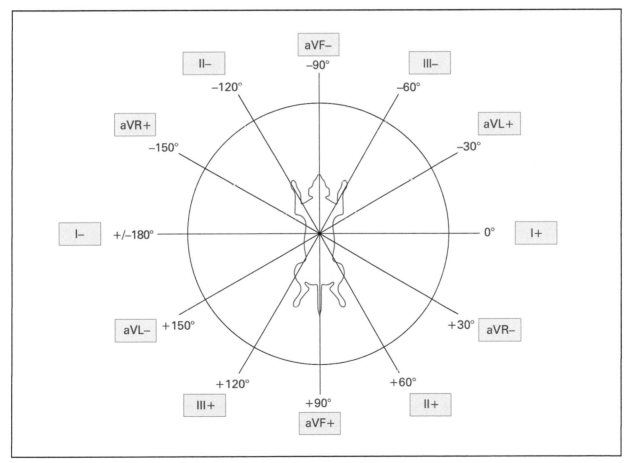

Fig. 2.4 The 6-lead ECG system.

and in the cat, the normal MEA is between 0 and +160 degrees (**Fig. 2.5**). An easy way to remember the direction of the normal MEA is to visualize a dorsoventral or ventrodorsal radiograph and imagine the normal MEA as pointing from the center of the heart toward the left ventricular apex. The MEA can be within the normal range or to the right or left of the normal range. Common causes of right axis deviation include right ventricular hypertrophy or right bundle branch block. A common cause of left axis deviation includes partial or incomplete bundle branch block. Note that left ventricular hypertrophy does not usually result in the left axis shift, as the normal MEA is already pointing in the direction of the left ventricular apex. Less commonly, mechanical displacement of the heart to either side of the thorax by space-occupying lesions or lung lobe atelectesis can change the MEA. Examples of animals with a left and right axis shift are shown in **Figure 2.6**.

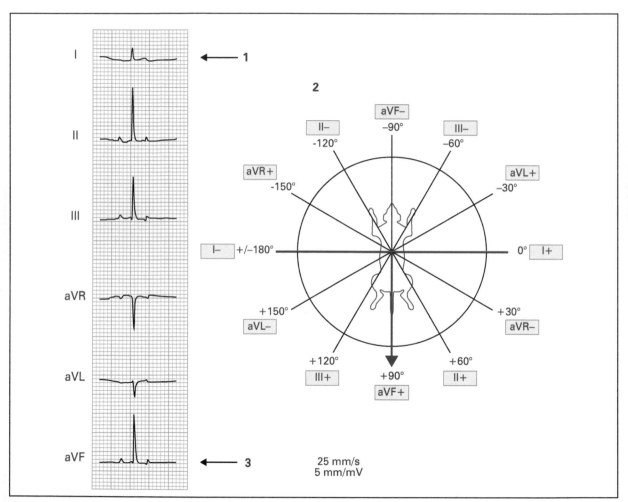

Fig. 2.5 Calculation of mean electrical axis (MEA). Calculation of the MEA is performed by examining the polarity of the QRS complexes from each of the six limb leads.

1. Identify the ECG lead in which the QRS complex is isoelectric, that is, the lead in which the net polarity of the QRS complex is closest to zero (i.e., the positive and negative deflections of the QRS waves cancel each other out). In some instances, this will be the lead in which the QRS waves are the smallest; and in other instances, the lead in which the amplitude of the positive QRS deflections is the same as the sum of the negative deflections. 2. Examine the hexaxial lead system and identify the limb lead that is perpendicular to the isoelectric lead. The MEA will exist in a direction either toward the positive or negative pole of the perpendicular lead.

3. Inspect the ECG and note the polarity of the QRS complex in the perpendicular lead.

4. If the net polarity is negative, the MEA points to the negative pole of the perpendicular lead; and if the net polarity is positive, the MEA points to the positive pole of the perpendicular lead.

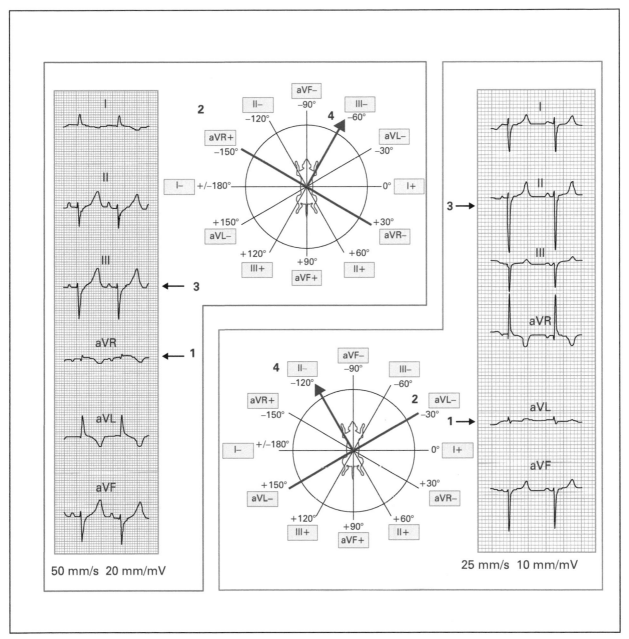

Fig. 2.6 Right shift (right panel) and left shift (left panel) in the mean electrical axis. See Figure 2.5 for numerals.

WAVEFORM MORPHOLOGY AND INTERVALS

The amplitudes, durations, and intervals of a representative normal P–QRS–T complex are shown in **Figure 2.7**.

The P wave

The P wave represents atrial depolarization. Increased P wave amplitude or duration is associated with either right and/or left atrial enlargement. Normal P wave values for the dog and cat are shown in *Table 2.1*. Absence of P waves is noted in instances of atrial fibrillation (AF), atrial standstill, and sinus arrest. P waves without corresponding QRS complexes are noted in cases of second- and third-degree AV node block. Inverted or retrograde P waves are commonly seen in conjunction with junctional or atrial premature and escape beats.

The PR interval

The PR interval represents the time it takes for the electrical impulse to conduct from the sinus node through the atria and the AV node and bundle of His. Physiologically, the delay in impulse conduction in the AV node allows the atria to empty of blood and for ventricular filling to occur, prior to the onset of ventricular contraction. The PR interval is measured from the start of the P wave to the first deflection of the QRS complex. The normal PR interval in dogs and cats is shown in Table 2.1. Increased duration of the PR interval is described as first-degree AV block. Varying PR intervals are noted in cases of sinus arrhythmia or certain forms of second-degree AV block. Abnormally short PR intervals are rare and encountered in instances of accessory pathway (AP)-mediated arrhythmias.

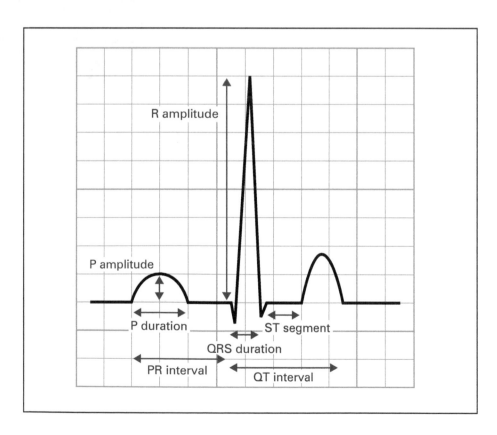

Fig. 2.7 Amplitudes, durations, and intervals of the P–QRS–T complex.

Evaluation of the Electrocardiogram

The QRS complex

The QRS complex represents ventricular depolarization. Standard nomenclature describes the first negative deflection as the Q wave, the first positive deflection as the R wave, and the first negative deflection following the first positive deflection as the S wave. Note that normal QRS complexes do not necessarily contain all three waveforms, and in dogs, a high degree of individual variability is seen. The normal sequence of ventricular depolarization results in a QRS complex of relatively short duration and with a net positive polarity in leads II, III, and aVF. The normal duration and amplitude of the QRS complex in the dog and cat is shown in Table 2.1. A key component of ECG analysis is inspection of the QRS morphology in lead II, which can provide clues to the complex's origin, its conduction through the ventricle, and the potential presence of ventricular hypertrophy. QRS complexes generated by a beat of supraventricular origin (sinus node or supraventricular foci such as the atria or AV nodal junction) are typically narrow and positive in lead II, while those that originate from ventricular foci are wider in duration and "bizarre" in their appearance as compared to normal sinus beats.

Conduction disturbances within the ventricles can also alter the morphology of the QRS complexes. Finally, ventricular hypertrophy can increase the amplitude of the QRS complex and the duration (albeit to a lesser degree than a bundle branch block) or change the MEA (as in the case of right heart enlargement, Fig. 2.6, p. 15).

Table 2.1 Normal ECG amplitude and duration in the dog and cat

	Dog	Cat
Heart rate	Puppy: 70–220 bpm Adult: 70–180 bpm	120–240 bpm
Rhythm	Sinus rhythm Sinus arrhythmia	Sinus rhythm
P wave		
Amplitude	Max: 0.4 mV	Max: 0.2 mV
Duration	Max: 0.04 s	Max: 0.04 s
PR interval	0.06–0.13 s	0.05–0.09 s
QRS		
Amplitude	Max: 2.5 mV, small breeds (3.0 mV, large breeds)	Max: 0.9 mV
Duration	≤0.06 s	≤0.04 s
ST segment	No elevation or depression >0.2 mV	No elevation or depression
T wave	Positive, negative, or biphasic, not >25% height or R wave	Isoelectric or usually positive and <0.3 mV
Electrical axis	+40° to +100°	0 to +160°

Source: Adapted from Tilley LP, Smith WK (2008). Electrocardiography. In: Tilley LP, Smith WK, Oyama MA, Sleeper MM (eds). *Manual of Canine and Feline Cardiology*, 4th edn. Saunders Elsevier, St Louis.

The ST segment

The ST segment (or interval) represents the time between the end of ventricular depolarization and the beginning of ventricular repolarization. In general, the ST segment should not be either elevated or depressed as compared to baseline by more than 0.2 mV. In human patients, ST segment abnormalities occur in instances of myocardial ischemia/infarction, pericardial disease, or electrolyte imbalances. In dogs and cats, ST segment abnormalities are occasionally detected in cases of myocardial disease (dilated cardiomyopathy), congenital heart disease (subaortic stenosis), electrolyte imbalances, acute hypoxia (anesthesia), or suspected myocardial infarction (rare).

The T wave

The T wave represents ventricular repolarization. The normal T wave in both dogs and cats demonstrates a high degree of variability and can be positive, negative, biphasic, or of very low amplitude; however, the T wave should be consistent from beat to beat during a normal rhythm. The normal characteristics of the T wave in dogs and cats are shown in Table 2.1. As compared to human patients, T wave changes in the dog and cat are relatively nonspecific and poorly characterized. T wave abnormalities can be seen in instances of electrolyte abnormalities, hypoxia, conduction abnormalities, or drug toxicity (i.e., digoxin). The duration of time from the start of the QRS complex to the end of the T wave is called the QT interval.

CRITERIA FOR HEART ENLARGEMENT

The criteria for heart enlargement in the dog and cat are shown in *Table 2.2*. In brief, left atrial enlargement is manifest as P wave of increased duration (P mitrale) or increased amplitude, and left ventricular enlargement as QRS waveforms with increased R wave amplitude and QRS duration. Right atrial enlargement is manifest as P waves of increased amplitude (P pulmonale) or increased duration, and right ventricular enlargement as a right MEA shift and prominent S waves. Examples of left and right heart enlargement patterns are shown in **Figures 2.8** and **2.9**.

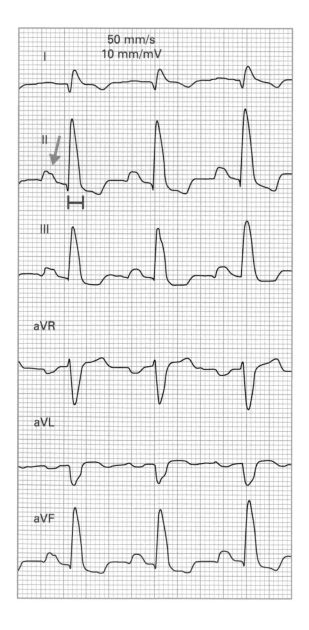

Fig. 2.8 Left atrial and ventricular enlargement in a dog is denoted by the wide and notched P wave (arrow) and wide QRS complex (red bar), respectively.

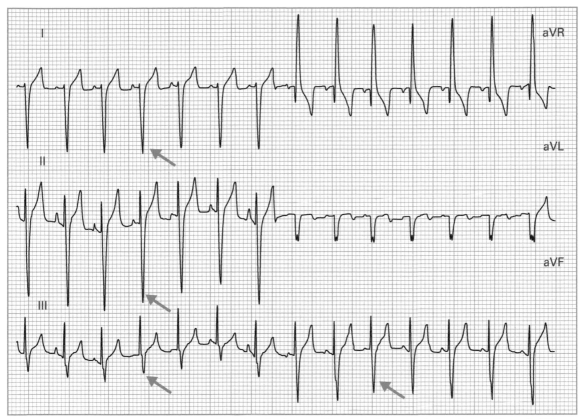

Fig. 2.9 Right ventricular enlargement in a dog is denoted by deep S waves in leads I, II, III, and aVF (arrows).

Table 2.2 ECG criteria for heart enlargement in the dog and cat

	Dog	Cat
Left atrial enlargement		
P wave	>0.4 mV	>0.04 s
	>0.04 s	
	Notched	
Right atrial enlargement		
P wave	>0.4 mV	>0.2 mV
Left ventricular enlargement		
R wave	>2.5 mV in lead II, aVF	>0.9 mV in lead II
	(>3.0 mV in large breed dogs)	
	>1.5 mV in lead I	
QRS duration*	>0.06 s	>0.04 s
Right ventricular enlargement		
S wave	>0.05 mV in lead I	S wave in leads I, II, III
	>0.35 mV in lead II	and aVF
Electrical axis	Right shift (>+100°)	Right shift (>+160°)

Source: Adapted from Tilley LP, Smith WK (2008). Electrocardiography. In: Tilley LP, Smith WK, Oyama MA, Sleeper MM (eds). *Manual of Canine and Feline Cardiology*, 4th edn. Saunders Elsevier, St Louis.

*QRS duration >0.08 s in the dog and >0.06 s in the cat can be associated with left or right bundle branch blocks. See text for more detail.

BUNDLE BRANCH BLOCK

The bundle of His is specialized conduction tissue that forms the distal portion of the AV node, and divides into two main bundle branches that course left- and rightward into the ventricular muscle. Right (RBBB) or left (LBBB) bundle branch block occurs when the impulse is blocked or slowed within either of the branches and block results in characteristic QRS waveform changes. In order to diagnose a bundle branch block, the MEA has to be determined, which requires a 6-lead ECG recording. RBBB is characterized by a right shift of the MEA and markedly prolonged QRS duration (>0.08 s in the dog and >0.06 s in the cat), while LBBB is characterized by a normal MEA and markedly prolonged QRS duration (>0.08 s in the dog and >0.06 s in the cat). Examples of RBBB and LBBB are shown in **Figures 2.10** and **2.11**. The wide QRS morphology of a bundle branch block pattern may be confused with a ventricular rhythm. Impulse origin in most cases of bundle branch block is the sinus node, hence there is a P wave associated with each QRS complex and the rhythm is supraventricular, despite the marked change in QRS waveform morphology. RBBB is typically a benign finding in both dogs and cats, whereas LBBB is usually associated with severe underlying heart disease.

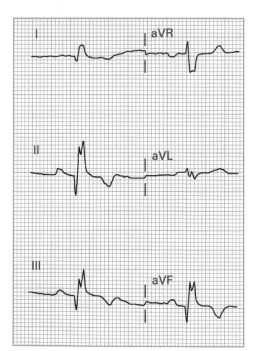 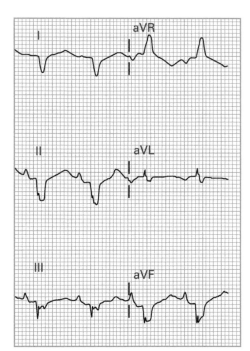

Figs. 2.10, 2.11 Bundle branch block. **Fig. 2.10**: Left bundle branch block in a dog. Note the presence of a P wave, the wide QRS complexes, and a normal mean electrical axis. **Fig. 2.11**: Right bundle branch block in a cat. Note the presence of the P wave, deep and wide S waves in leads I, II, III, and aVF, and the right mean electrical axis deviation.

Section 3

APPROACH TO EVALUATING ARRHYTHMIAS

Cardiac arrhythmias are defined as variations of the cardiac rhythm from normal sinus rhythm (too rapid, too slow, or too irregular). "Ectopic" beats are those that arise from a source other than the sinus node. Some cardiac arrhythmias are benign and clinically insignificant and require no therapy, whereas other arrhythmias are malignant and potentially life-threatening (i.e., ventricular tachycardia [VT] or ventricular fibrillation [VF]) causing clinical signs such as weakness, lethargy, syncope, or sudden death.

Although a specific diagnosis may be suggested by auscultation (i.e., AF, high-grade AV block) and physical examination, an ECG is required for a definitive diagnosis.

SYSTEMIC APPROACH TO RHYTHM DIAGNOSIS

Questions to ask:
- Is the rate fast or slow (tachycardia *vs.* bradycardia)?
- Is the rhythm regular or irregular? If irregular, is the rate slow, fast, or are there premature beats?
- Are there P waves? Are they normal (upright in lead II – i.e., is the rhythm sinus or not sinus) (**Fig. 3.1**)?
- Is there a P wave for every QRS; is there a QRS for every P wave?
- Are the QRS complexes normal or abnormal (normal or abnormal conduction)?

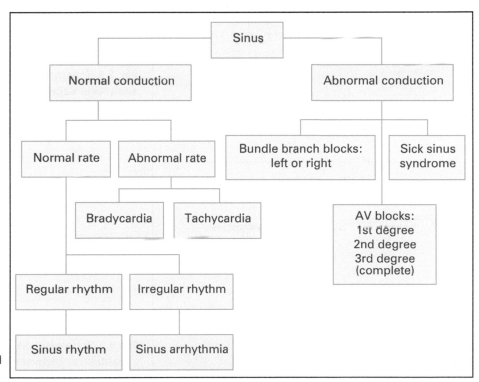

Fig. 3.1 Schematic diagram of rhythm analysis in sinus rhythm (P waves have to be present to be considered a sinus rhythm).

HOW DOES ONE DIFFERENTIATE SUPRAVENTRICULAR ARRHYTHMIAS FROM VENTRICULAR ARRHYTHMIAS?

Supraventricular arrhythmias: General criteria (**Fig. 3.2**):

- Ectopic beats display a narrow QRS complex.
- Morphology of ectopic QRS complexes and sinus beat QRS complexes are similar.
- P waves usually associated with the ectopic QRS (unless heart rate is rapid enough so that the P waves are buried within the preceding T wave or if AF or atrial flutter [AFL] are present).
- P wave morphology of ectopic beats can appear different from the sinus P wave.

Ventricular arrhythmias: General criteria (**Fig. 3.3**):

- Wide QRS complex.
- Morphology of ectopic QRS complexes and sinus beat QRS complexes are dissimilar.
- P waves are not associated with the ectopic QRS complex.
- If fusion beats are present, this supports a diagnosis of ventricular ectopic complexes.

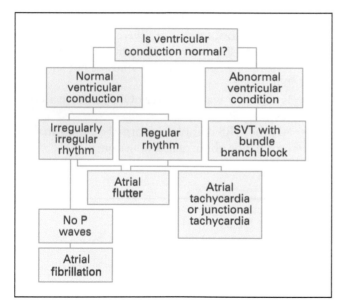

Fig. 3.2 Schematic diagram of rhythm analysis in supraventricular arrhythmias. SVT: supraventricular tachycardia.

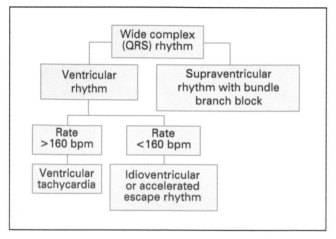

Fig. 3.3 Schematic diagram of rhythm analysis in ventricular tachycardia (wide QRS complex rhythm).

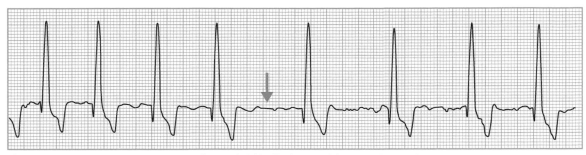

Fig. 3.4 Dog, lead II, 50 mm/s showing atrial fibrillation and f waves (arrow).

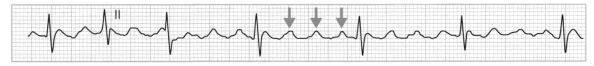

Fig. 3.5 Dog, lead II, 50 mm/s showing atrial flutter and Fl waves (arrows).

SUPRAVENTRICULAR ARRHYTHMIAS

Supraventricular arrhythmias (SVAs) originate in the sinus node, atrial tissue, and AV junction (or AV node). SVAs include a wide variety of atrial, AV junction, and AV nodal tachycardias. SVAs have to be differentiated from sinus tachycardia. Sinus tachycardia is typically physiological and may be caused by many conditions including febrile states, anemia, heart failure, adrenergic medications, and anxiety.

Specific supraventricular arrhythmias and ECG criteria

Atrial fibrillation

AF is caused by multiple atrial impulses that depolarize the atria simultenously and bombard the AV node. During AF, the atrial activation rate is rapid and can exceed 500 depolarizations/minute. The refractory period of the AV node does not allow all these impulses to travel to the ventricle, and prevents heart rates exceeding 250–300 bpm. This protects the ventricles from developing VF as a consequence of AF. The electrophysiological mechanisms that initiate and maintain AF include abnormal automaticity and re-entry.

ECG criteria (**Fig. 3.4**):
- P waves are absent.
- Atrial activity is represented by fibrillatory (f) waves of varying amplitudes.
- Irregular ventricular rhythm.
- At very rapid rates the rhythm can appear more regular.

Most cases of AF in small animals are associated with significant underlying heart disease. In giant breed dogs, AF can occur spontaneously, and in the absence of identifiable heart disease, the term "lone" AF is often used.

Atrial flutter

AFL is a form of re-entry tachycardia that usually arises from the right atrium. It utilizes the anatomy of the right atrium to sustain a macro-re-entry loop of continuous depolarization. It can also be initiated and sustained in the left atrium. It is maintained due to differences in the refractory periods of atrial tissue. As in AF, the AV node controls the ventricular response rate.

ECG criteria (**Fig. 3.5**):
- Rapid ventricular rate possible.
- Sawtooth undulation of the baseline.
- Atrial (f wave) rate usually >300 bpm.
- Rate and regularity of RR intervals can be variable (depends on AV conduction). Often 2:1 or 3:1 conduction patterns are observed.

Focal (ectopic) atrial tachycardia

Focal atrial tachycardia (FAT) occurs when localized regions in the atria (other than the sinus or AV node) develop the ability to fire rapidly on their own. Depending on the site of the focus, the morphology of the P wave observed on the surface ECG varies. On occasion, multifocal atrial tachycardia can develop, in which case the P wave morphology varies depending on the shifting atrial focus. The electrophysiological mechanisms that initiate and maintain FAT include abnormal automaticity, re-entry, and triggered activity.

ECG criteria (**Fig. 3.6**):
- Normal P waves or abnormal P waves that are different in morphology from sinus P waves.
- There may be a "warm-up" period observed where the heart rate gradually accelerates after initiation of the tachycardia.
- Atrial rate generally >180 bpm.
- The ventricular rhythm may be irregular when the atrial rate is so rapid that not every atrial beat is conducted to the ventricles (physiological second-degree AV block).

Atrioventricular re-entrant tachycardia

Atrioventricular re-entrant tachycardia (AVRT) is a macro-re-entry arrhythmia whose circuit comprises the AV node as well as an accessory pathway (AP) which can conduct impulses between the atrial and ventricles, often time in either direction, thus bypassing the AV node and His–Purkinje system. During typical AVRT, the depolarization proceeds from the atria to the ventricles through the AV node, and back up to the atria from the ventricles in the retrograde direction via the AP. An AP can behave like a two-way street for electric conduction. If during normal sinus rhythm, early activation (pre-excitation) of the ventricle occurs via atrial to ventricular conduction along the AP, a delta wave (slurring of the upstroke of the QRS complex) on the surface ECG can occur. Some APs can only conduct in the retrograde direction and therefore do not show a pre-excitation pattern.

ECG criteria:
- Short PR interval (if the impulse is transmitted forward from atria to ventricle over the AP).
- Delta wave (if the impulse is transmitted forward from atria to ventricle over the AP).
- During typical AVRT, QRS complexes are usually narrow and the retrograde P wave (negative polarity in leads II and III) may be seen embedded into the early portion of the T wave.

- One-to-one atrial to ventricular association is usually present during AVRT because the atria and ventricles are both integral parts of the arrhythmia circuit.

BRADYARRHYTHMIAS AND CONDUCTION DISTURBANCES
Sinus bradycardia

Sinus bradycardia (SB) is a type of sinus rhythm where the sinus node discharge rate is low (<50 bpm in an awake dog). SB of 45–60 bpm during sleep is normal. However, if SB persists during excitement or exercise, it can be a sign of sinus node pathology.

ECG criteria (**Fig. 3.7**):
- Sinus rhythm with positive P waves in the caudal leads (II, III, aVF) and normal QRS complexes, unless concurrent conduction disease is present.
- Slow sinus node discharge rate.
- Escape beats (junctional or ventricular) may be present.

SICK SINUS SYNDROME

Sick sinus syndrome (SSS) is a disease process in which the spontaneous sinus node discharge is either slower than normal (primary SB) or intermittently absent (sinus arrest or sinus block). It is characterized by an atrial rate that is inappropriate for a patient's activity. The subsidiary pacemaker tissue (AV node and Purkinje fibers) is often also abnormal, resulting in inadequate escape rhythms, such that complete asystole (pauses) can occur, often lasting many seconds. Clinical signs associated with SSS may include fainting or intermittent weakness. Some patients experience supraventricular tachycardia (SVT) as well as bradycardia or sinus arrest.

ECG criteria (**Fig. 3.8**):
- The ECG demonstrates a collection of conditions that indicate sinus node and escape rhythm dysfunction.
- Periods of bradycardia or sinus arrest followed by paroxysms of SVT.
- AV block may also be present.
- Due to the intermittent nature of the arrhythmia, 24-hour ambulatory ECG (Holter) monitoring is often necessary to diagnose this condition definitively.

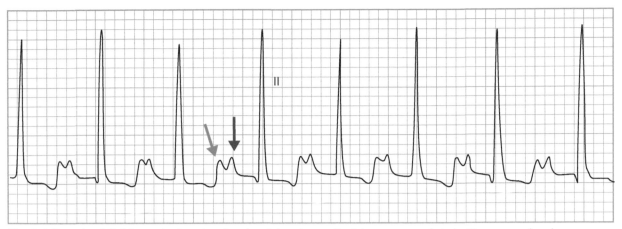

Fig. 3.6 Dog, lead II, 25 mm/s showing focal atrial tachycardia (blue arrow points to T wave and red arrow points to P wave).

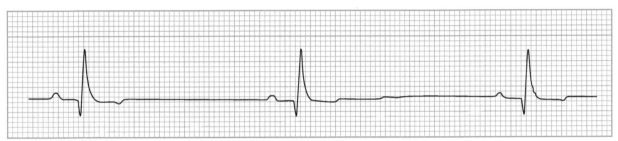

Fig. 3.7 Dog, lead aVF, 50 mm/s showing sinus bradycardia, with a heart rate of 65 bpm.

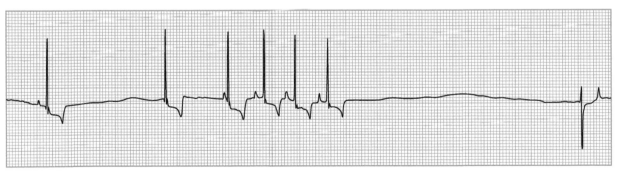

Fig. 3.8 Dog, lead II, 25 mm/s showing sick sinus syndrome, with a period of sinus arrest and junctional (second beat from the left) and ventricular (last beat on the right) escape beats.

ATRIAL STANDSTILL

Atrial standstill is a lack of electrocardiographic evidence of atrial depolarization, resulting in the absence of P waves on the ECG. Causes include hyperkalemia, digitalis toxicity, and primary atrial myocardial disease.

ECG criteria (**Fig. 3.9**):
- No P waves are present.
- Slow junctional or ventricular escape rhythm is often present.
- If associated with hyperkalemia, the T waves can be tall and the QRS morphology can be wide and bizarre.

AV CONDUCTION ABNORMALITIES (AV BLOCK)

AV block consists of incomplete, intermittent, or complete failure of conduction between the atria and ventricles via the AV node. Three types of AV block exist:
- First-degree AV block (**Fig. 3.10**) is defined as prolonged conduction through the AV node that results in an increased PR interval of >0.13 s (dog) and >0.09 s (cat) and normal P wave and QRS complexes, in a 1:1 ratio.
- Second-degree AV block (**Fig. 3.11**) is a conduction disorder in which some atrial impulses are not conducted to the ventricles. There are normal P waves and QRS complexes, but intermittently the P waves are not followed by QRS complexes (blocked P). Second-degree AV block occurs in two types:

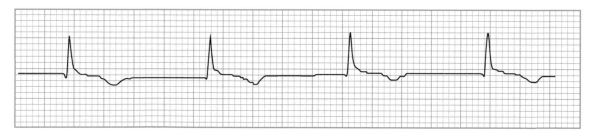

Fig. 3.9 Cat, lead aVL, 50 mm/s showing atrial standstill.

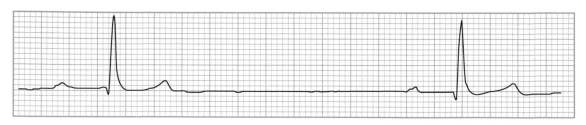

Fig. 3.10 Dog, lead II, 50 mm/s showing first-degree atrioventricular block, with a PR interval of 0.16 s.

- Mobitz type I (Wenckebach) AV block: PR interval gradually prolongs until conduction across the AV node fails, hence no QRS complex occurs following the P (dropped beat).
- Mobitz type II AV block: The PR interval is usually constant before a dropped beat occurs. This is considered a more advanced form of block that occurs lower in the His bundle and may thus progress to complete heart block.
- In third-degree (complete) AV block (**Fig. 3.12**), none of the P waves conduct through the AV node, thus the atrial and ventricular activities are completely independent (AV dissociation). The atrial rate is faster than the ventricular rate. The escape rhythm is either junctional or ventricular in origin.

VENTRICULAR ARRHYTHMIAS

Ventricular arrhythmias are abnormal spontaneous depolarizations that originate in any location in the ventricle. The occurrence of three or more ventricular premature contractions (VPCs) in a row is termed VT. Descriptions of ventricular arrhythmias often include whether or not the morphology of all VPCs is similar (monomorphic) or different (polymorphic), occurs as a single VPC, two VPCs in a row (couplet), or three or more VPCs in a row (VT). Furthermore, a period of VT is often described as persisting less than 30 seconds (nonsustained) or more than 30 seconds (sustained). Breed-specific ventricular arrhythmias occur especially in Boxers, Doberman Pinschers, and German Shepherd dogs. An analysis algorithm for differentiation of wide QRS complex arrhythmias is shown in Figure 3.3 p. 22.

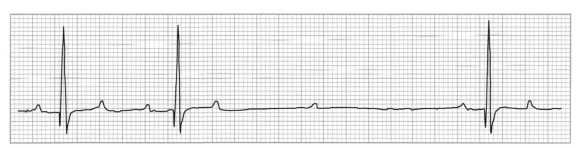

Fig. 3.11 Dog, lead II, 50 mm/s showing second-degree atrioventricular block, with a blocked P wave seen in the middle of the strip.

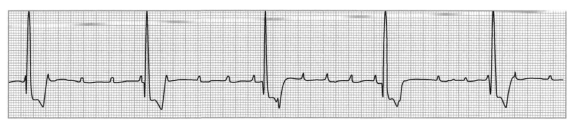

Fig. 3.12 Dog, lead II, 25 mm/s showing third-degree atrioventricular block.

ECG criteria (**Figs. 3.13, 3.14**):
- Abnormally wide and bizarre QRS complexes as compared to the normal sinus QRS complex.
- No associated P waves.
- Rate of ventricular beats is similar to (AV dissociation) or greater than the P wave rate (VT).
- Fusion beats are often present.

VENTRICULAR FIBRILLATION

Ventricular fibrillation (VF) is an irregular chaotic rhythm during which there is no organized ventricular contraction. VF is a fatal arrhythmia because it is never self-terminating and is associated with little to no cardiac output. Electric defibrillation is the only viable treatment option.

ECG criteria (**Fig. 3.15**):
- Chaotic and irregular deflections of varying amplitudes.
- No distinguishable P, QRS, or T waves are present.

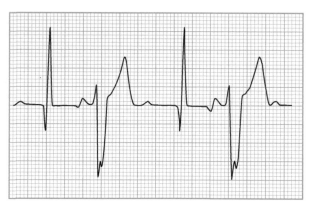

Fig. 3.13 Dog, lead II, 50 mm/s showing ventricular premature beats.

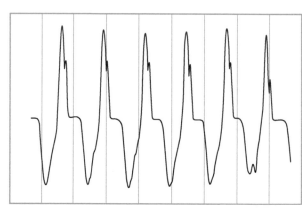

Fig. 3.14 Dog, lead II, 50 mm/s showing ventricular tachycardia.

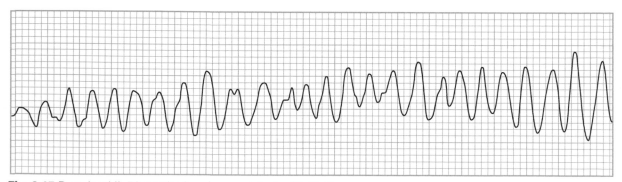

Fig. 3.15 Dog, lead II, 50 mm/s showing ventricular fibrillation.

Section 4

TREATMENT OF ARRHYTHMIAS

The decision on whether or not and how to treat arrhythmias depends on factors such as a history of collapse, the heart rate during an arrhythmia, the presence and severity of underlying heart disease, and affected dog breed (predispositions of most commonly affected breeds; for genetic VT abnormalities, see Box 4.1), as well as the presence of various systemic diseases that potentially contribute to the presence of arrhythmias.

Therapy of arrhythmias should not be instituted without an ECG to provide a definitive diagnosis of the nature of the arrhythmia. By auscultation alone, some ventricular arrhythmias can be confused with supraventricular arrhythmias such as atrial tachycardia or atrial fibrillation, which warrant very different treatment strategies. Ambulatory, long-term ECG recordings, such as 24-hour Holter monitoring, might be required to establish a definitive diagnosis since many arrhythmias are intermittent and might not be documented during a short in-hospital ECG. (See Section 5 for Holter monitoring.) Post-treatment 24-hour Holter recordings are highly useful for assessment of drug efficacy, and also allow for detection of drug toxicity, such as proarrhythmia (worsening ventricular arrhythmias) or drug overdose, for instance, bradycardia or pauses secondary to excessive AV block. Pauses, if they occur only during sleep or rest, are usually of low concern.

In addition to medical therapy, interventional techniques, such as radiofrequency ablation, are a potentially curative treatment of certain supraventricular arrhythmias (AFL, AVRT), but are only offered at certain veterinary specialty clinics.

Cardiac arrhythmias in cats most commonly are associated with underlying heart disease, such as HCM or RCM, where sudden cardiac death is thought to be linked to the presence of complex arrhythmias. Arrhythmias can also occur secondary to systemic disease, namely hyperthyroidism, electrolyte imbalances (i.e., hyperkalemia), feline aortic thromboembolism, anemia, neoplasia, or drug reactions, in which case therapy should be aimed at correcting or managing the underlying disease. Cats of any breed, age, or sex may experience arrhythmias but Maine Coon cats are predisposed to HCM and thus commonly reported to have arrhythmias. Single VPCs and APCs are most commonly found on Holter recordings of cats with HCM, but complex arrhythmias with sustained VT and SVT are also reported, while healthy cats rarely show any ectopic beats. Occasionally, cats are diagnosed with atrial fibrillation. Typically, these cats have advanced underlying heart disease with marked dilation of the atria.

Clinical signs of arrhythmias are often hard to identify in cats, with lethargy or collapse being most suggestive of a possible arrhythmia. Congestive heart failure, aortic thromboembolism or signs of hyperthyroidism should prompt a careful evaluation for arrhythmias as a sequalae to the primary disease process, as this population is at greatest risk for sudden death. Due to the cats poor tolerance for wearing Holters, most arrhythmias are monitored by ECG only.

MECHANISMS OF ANTIARRHYTHMIC DRUGS

Antiarrhythmic drugs target two general areas of the heart because of their specific electrophysiologic properties:

1. *Sinoatrial (SA) and AV nodal tissue:*
   Depolarization in these tissues is calcium-channel driven and sensitive to autonomic tone. To treat arrhythmias that originate from the SA and AV nodal tissue, calcium-channel blockers (CCBs) and beta-blockers (BBs) are primarily used. The most commonly prescribed CCB for treatment of arrhythmias is diltiazem (available PO and IV). The β1-selective BBs atenolol and esmolol (IV only) are the most frequently

Box 4.1 Breed-specific arrhythmias

Breed	Genetics	ECG characteristics	Comments
Boxers	• ARVC is inherited as autosomal dominant trait with adult onset of disease • Some Boxers have a mutation in the striatin gene with incomplete penetrance	• VPCs and VT common • The typical VPC QRS morphology is a left bundle branch block pattern (i.e., QRS in leads II, III, and aVF are predominantly positive) • A subset of Boxers may experience bradycardia-associated syncope due to sinus arrest or sinus bradycardia	• Boxers with the striatin mutation variably express clinical disease and it is likely that there is more than one ARVC mutation in Boxers • Striatin is a desmosomal protein (scaffolding protein) located in the intercalated disc region of the cardiomyocyte. DNA testing is available • Homozygous dogs are more likely to have clinical signs and should not be used for breeding • Syncope is the most common presenting sign • Usually present at 4–6 years of age, and frequency and severity of the arrhythmia usually increase over time
English Bulldog	• Inherited ARVC • Genetic mode of inheritance is undetermined	• Similar to that of the Boxer with ARVC • VT and sudden death in 13% of dogs	• There is 2.9:1 male to female ratio of affectedness • Unlike Boxers with ARVC, the majority of English Bulldogs present with signs of CHF at the time of arrhythmia detection • Mean age of 9.2 years at time of presentation for arrhythmias
Doberman Pinschers	• Dilated cardiomyopathy (DCM) with ventricular arrhythmias in Doberman Pinschers inherited as autosomal dominant trait with adult onset of disease • At least two genetic mutations, one of which involves pyruvate dehydrogenase kinase 4 (PDK4), which is associated with mitochondrial alterations; DM2 is a titin abnormality	• VPCs and VT common • The typical VPC QRS morphology is a right bundle branch block pattern (i.e., QRS in leads II, III, and aVF are predominantly negative) • VPC and VT can be either monomorphic or polymorphic • Holter recording results indicating ≥1 VPC/hr, or ≥50 VPC/24 hours, or ≥1 couplet or triplet/24 hours are highly suggestive of DCM	• Doberman Pinschers with genetic mutations variably express clinical disease, and it is likely that there is more than one DCM mutation in Doberman Pinschers • Sudden death occurs in 30%–50% of affected dogs and is presumed to be caused by VT leading to ventricular fibrillation

(Continued)

Box 4.1 (*Continued*) Breed-specific arrhythmias

Breed	Genetics	ECG characteristics	Comments
English Springer Spaniels	• Mutation in the *KCNQ1* (Ware et al. 2015) gene	• Prolonged QT duration • QT>260–270 msec; QTc> 304–314 msec • T wave morphology is biphasic	• Defect of a repolarizing K$^+$ channel • Risk of sudden death
German Shepherds	• Inherited VT • Inheritance is polygenic due to an abnormality in a major gene with modifiers	• Large variation in ECG findings ranging from few VPCs to sustained and rapid polymorphic VT	• There are no identifiable gross abnormalities; disease involves the ion channels, resulting in repolarization abnormalities • Ventricular arrhythmias develop at 12–16 weeks of age, and the frequency and severity of the arrhythmias increase until 24–30 weeks of age • After 8 months of age, the arrhythmia severity stabilizes or starts to decrease • Risk of sudden death correlates with severity of the arrhythmia
Rhodesian Ridgebacks (Meurs et al. 2016)	• Ventricular arrhythmias inherited in an autosomal recessive mode and linked to mutations in the *QIL1* gene, which is involved in mitochondrial function	• VPCs and VT • In some dogs, atrial premature beats and second-degree AV nodal block present • No QT interval prolongation	• Dogs can remain free of clinical signs; however, sudden death can occur, usually before 1 year of age • There are no identifiable gross abnormalities

used antiarrhythmic BBs. Digoxin has a mild vagomimetic effect and can indirectly contribute to prolonging AV node conduction time; however, its antiarrhythmic utility is primarily limited to the treatment of AF.

2. *Atrial or ventricular myocardium:*
Depolarization in these tissues is sodium-channel driven, and repolarization primarily involves the potassium channel. To treat arrhythmias that originate from the atrial and ventricular myocardium, sodium-channel blockers, potassium-channel blockers, or combinations thereof are often used in conjunction with BBs. The sodium-channel blockers commonly used for treatment of arrhythmias in dogs are lidocaine (IV only), mexiletine, and, rarely, procainamide. The most important potassium-channel blocker is sotalol, which also has BB properties. Amiodarone, which is predominantly a potassium-channel blocker but also has potent sodium-channel blocker and some CCB and BB activity, is occasionally used for arrhythmias that are particularly difficult to control.

TREATMENT OF ARRHYTHMIAS
Treatment of supraventricular arrhythmias

Supraventricular arrhythmias (SVA) include rhythms that originate in the sinus node, atrial tissue, and AV junction. Physiologic sinus tachycardia must be differentiated from SVA and is typically caused by systemic disease states associated with fever, anemia, heart failure, adrenergic medications, or anxiety and pain. As such, correcting the underlying cause can result in normalization of the heart rate.

The decision regarding how and when to treat a supraventricular arrhythmia is based on presence and frequency of the clinical signs, such as fainting or co-existing congestive heart failure. Emergency management using intravenous drugs may be indicated before a 24-hour Holter recording can be obtained. Both diltiazem and esmolol are available in an IV formulation, allowing emergency treatment of very rapid supraventricular arrhythmias. See *Table 4.1* for drugs commonly used in the treatment of supraventricular arrhythmias.

Atrial fibrillation (AF)

Treatment of AF largely depends on the heart rate (i.e., ventricular response rate). Conversion of AF to sinus rhythm with antiarrhythmic drugs is rarely achieved in dogs and never even attempted in cats.

In most cases, ventricular rate control via slowing of AV node conduction with diltiazem and or digoxin is the primary goal (Table 4.1). For clinically unstable dogs (i.e., those with overt weakness, syncope, or congestive heart failure [CHF]) and/or those with HR >250 bpm, IV therapy to slow the ventricular response quickly, using diltiazem IV bolus, followed by a constant-rate infusion and subsequent titration to oral medications, is often performed.

In clinically stable dogs with AF, oral therapy is started using diltiazem and digoxin. Extended-release diltiazem (Dilacor-XR) has the advantage of twice daily dosing over diltiazem modified release, which requires 3 times daily dosing. An effect on HR typically occurs within a few hours of oral dosing. Only mild effects on contractility are seen with diltiazem when given at prescribed doses. Diltiazem is often co-administered with digoxin. Atenolol can also be used, but due to its potential to decrease contractility, particularly in dogs with poor systolic function or in heart failure, initial doses should be relatively low and then subsequently titrated as needed. The electrocardiographic goal of chronic AF therapy is a 24-hour-average heart rate of <125 bpm as determined by post-treatment Holter recordings. Rate control for AF in cats is attempted with dilacor-XR monotherapy (for drug dosages, see Table 4.1). Due to poor bioavailability the oral dose is much higher in cats than in dogs.

Dogs with AF but little to no underlying heart disease (often referred to as "primary" or "lone" AF) are candidates for electric cardioversion of AF to sinus rhythm while under anesthesia.

Electrical cardioversion refers to a synchronized delivery of an electrical shock to the heart, which depolarizes the majority of the cardiac muscle at one time. The myocardium becomes temporarily inexcitable, causing disruption of the AF, thus promoting the return of sinus rhythm. Shock delivery must be timed with the QRS complex (i.e., synchronized) to avoid delivery during the vulnerable T wave segment, which could induce ventricular fibrillation. Cardioversion units will possess a synchronization feature (SYNC) that must be used with the supplied ECG leads. Newer defibrillators deliver biphasic shocks, which improve effectiveness at lower energy levels compared with the older monophasic units.

Dogs with primary AF typically have lower ventricular response rates than dogs with underlying heart disease and are often asymptomatic. One advantage of cardioversion even in cases of

Table 4.1 Drugs for treatment of supraventricular arrhythmias

Drug	Administration per os	Parenteral administration	Comments
Diltiazem HCl (Cardizem); (Extended release: Dilacor XR)	*Dog:* 0.5–2 mg/kg TID Dilacor XR: 2.5–4.5 mg/kg BID *Cat:* Dilacor XR: 30–60 mg/cat SID to BID	*Dog:* 0.05–0.25 mg/kg IV bolus followed by CRI: 2–6 µg/kg/min *Cat:* 0.1–0.4 mg/kg, IV bolus over ~1 minute followed by CRI: Titrate to effect 2–6 µg/kg/min	Intravenous dosing can cause transient hypotension and AV nodal block
Digoxin	*Dog:* 0.0025–0.0035 mg/kg BID (or 0.11 mg/m^2 BID) *Cat:* 0.03125 mg/cat every other day		Do not exceed 0.25 mg per dog BID
Procainamide		*Dog:* 5–15 mg/kg IV bolus slowly over 2 minutes, CRI: 25–50 µg/kg/min	Can decrease contractility
Esmolol HCl		*Dog and cat:* 50–100 µg/kg IV bolus, repeat up to max 500 µg/kg CRI: Titrate to effect: 50–200 µg/kg/min	Can decrease contractility; can combine with any other IV antiarrhythmic; use with caution in combination with procainamide
Atenolol	*Dog:* 0.5–2 mg/kg SID to BID *Cat:* 6.25–12 mg SID to BID		Titrate to effect; can decrease contractility
Amiodarone	*Dog:* 5–15 mg/kg BID for 1–2 weeks (loading dose), then 6–15 mg/kg SID (maintenance dose)	*Dog:* 2 mg/kg IV bolus slowly over 10 min CRI: 0.8 mg/kg/h for 6 h, the 0.4 mg/kg/h	Can combine with atenolol for refractory supraventricular tachycardia Aqueous (water-based) formulations are better tolerated than polysorbate 80/alcohol-based formulations
Sotalol	*Dog:* 1.5–2.5 mg/kg BID *Cat:* 10 mg/cat BID		

Abbreviations: CRI, continuous rate infusion; IV, intravenous.

primary AF is avoidance of structural or functional myocardial remodeling that results secondary to chronic AF. Recurrence of AF after cardioversion is unpredictable. Pre-treatment with amiodarone or sotalol may improve the chances of successful cardioversion.

Atrial flutter (AFL)

Treatment of AFL is similar to treatment of AF, and ventricular rate control via slowing of the AV node with a CCB or BB is commonly performed (for drug dosages, see treatment for AF and Table 4.1). Medical conversion of AFL to sinus rhythm with antiarrhythmic drugs such as a potassium-channel blocker (sotalol) is rarely achieved in dogs. Radiofrequency ablation has been used successfully in a small number of dogs.

Focal (ectopic) atrial tachycardia (FAT)

Ideally, the rapidly firing atrial focus, which is the underlying mechanism, is suppressed using sotalol, amiodarone, or procainamide (see Table 4.1). However, similar to AF and AFL, slowing of AV node conduction with a CCB or BB can be used either with or without these drugs to reduce the ventricular response rate. Digoxin is usually ineffective for management of FAT.

Atrioventricular re-entry tachycardia (AVRT)

Treatment of AVRT, especially in animals with syncope, lethargy, or congestive heart failure, typically involves a CCB or BB. For acute management of dogs with incessant tachycardia, intravenous diltiazem or esmolol is commonly administered, followed by titration to oral dosing.

Oral sotalol, procainamide, or amiodarone is often co-administered in order to slow conduction in the atria, accessory pathways, and ventricles. In dogs with drug-refractory AVRT and clinical signs, radiofrequency ablation should be considered.

Treatment of bradyarrhythmias

Clinically significant bradyarrhythmias that typically require treatment involve sinus node dysfunction (e.g., sinus bradycardia or sick sinus syndrome [SSS]), atrial standstill, or AV node conduction abnormalities (e.g., high-grade, second-degree or third-degree AV block). Drugs commonly used to treat bradyarrhythmias are listed in *Table 4.2*.

Sinus bradycardia

Sinus bradycardia, beyond what occurs because of normal vagal tone, can be due to conduction system disease (i.e., SSS) or secondary to an underlying systemic disease (i.e., Addison's disease), electrolyte abnormalities (i.e., hyperkalemia), drug toxicity (e.g., narcotics or overdosing of BBs, CCBs), or excessively increased vagal tone (i.e., secondary to gastrointestinal or central nervous system disease). Correction of the underlying condition or discontinuation of drugs may resolve secondary sinus bradycardia. Animals that are syncopal due to bradycardia most likely require pacemaker therapy, as oral drugs are not effective at accelerating the heart rate. If immediate pacemaker therapy is not an option, medical therapy can be attempted. An atropine response test can help identify patients that would benefit from such medical management. Following injection of atropine IM or IV, the baseline heart rate should increase by 50%–100% within 5–10 minutes (initial worsening of AV block is a normal transient response). Patients experiencing at least a partial response to atropine may be candidates for medical management of sinus bradycardia. Treatment options include either vagolytics (e.g., probantheline bromide), sympathomimetics (e.g., terbulatine), or a phosphodiesterase inhibitor (e.g., theophylline); for drug doses, see *Table 4.3*. In animals with no clinical signs, sinus bradycardia might be "waited out" with close monitoring.

Sick sinus syndrome (SSS)

Most dogs with SSS exhibit clinical signs ranging from exercise intolerance and lethargy (which may be under-recognized by owners and mistakenly attributed to aging) to frequent syncope. If clinical signs are intermittent, 24-hour Holter recordings are often necessary to attribute the signs to SSS. Pacemaker therapy is typically required for syncopal or lethargic dogs with SSS. In animals without syncope or with no, or only mild, clinical signs, watchful waiting or medical management can be attempted (see medical treatment of sinus bradycardia).

Table 4.2 Drugs for treatment of bradyarrhythmias

Drug	Administration per os	Intravenous administration	Comments
Atropine sulfate		*Dog and cat:* 0.02–0.04 mg/kg IV bolus or IM	Can cause transient worsening of AV nodal block
Probantheline bromide	*Dog:* 0.25–5 mg/kg BID to TID *Cat:* 0.25–0.5 mg/kg or 7.5 mg/cat BID to TID		Can cause mydriasis, constipation, dry mouth, keratoconjunctivitis sicca
Terbutaline	*Dog:* 1.25–5 mg/dog BID to TID *Cat:* 0.312–1.25 mg/cat BID to TID		
Theophylline	*Dog:* 10–20 mg/kg BID *Cat:* 15–25 mg/kg SID		Can cause restlessness and anxiety, panting, nausea, vomiting, diarrhea, polydipsia, polyuria

Abbreviations: IV, intravenous; IM, intramuscular.

Table 4.3 Drugs for treatment of ventricular arrhythmias

Drug	Administration per os	Intravenous administration	Comments
Lidocaine		*Dog:* 2 mg/kg IV bolus, repeat up to 4 times CRI: 30–75 µg/kg/min *Cat:* 0.25–2 mg/kg IV bolus slowly CRI: 10–40 µg/kg/min	Cats have low seizure threshold
Procainamide		*Dog:* 5–15 mg/kg IV bolus slowly over 2 minutes CRI: 25–50 µg/kg/min	Can decrease contractility
Amiodarone	*Dog:* 5–15 mg/kg BID for 1–2 weeks (loading dose), then 6–15 mg/kg SID (maintenance dose)	Dog: 2 mg/kg IV bolus slowly over 10 min CRI: 0.8 mg/kg/h for 6 h, then 0.4 mg/kg/h	Can combine with atenolol for refractory ventricular tachycardia; aqueous (water-based) formulations are better tolerated than polysorbate 80/alcohol-based formulations
Esmolol HCl		*Dog and cat:* 50–100 µg/kg IV bolus, repeat up to max 500 µg/kg CRI: Titrate to effect: 50–200 µg/kg/min	Can decrease contractility; can combine with any other IV antiarrhythmic; use with caution in combination with procainamide
Sotalol	*Dog:* 1.5–2.5 mg/kg BID *Cat:* 10 mg/cat BID		Can combine with mexiletine for refractory ventricular tachycardia; also useful if IV drugs fail, as effect after oral dosing starts within 2–3 hours
Mexiletine	*Dog:* 4–8 mg/kg TID		Not effective as monotherapy
Atenolol	*Dog:* 0.5–2 mg/kg SID to BID *Cat:* 6.25–12 mg SID to BID		Titrate to effect; can decrease contractility; can combine with mexiletine for refractory ventricular tachycardia

Abbreviations: CRI, continuous rate infusion; IV, intravenous

Atrial standstill

The two main types are (1) persistent atrial standstill or "silent atrium" due to primary atrial muscle disease and (2) secondary atrial standstill caused by hyperkalemia secondary to diseases such as renal failure, ruptured bladder, or Addison's disease. If atrial muscle disease is causing atrial standstill, pacemaker therapy is required. For atrial standstill secondary to hyperkalemia, IV fluids, such as saline, half-strength saline with 2.5% dextrose, or 5% dextrose in water, will lower potassium values by dilution and increased excretion. The dextrose in fluid therapy leads to insulin secretion, which promotes entry of K^+ ions back into the cells. More aggressive therapy involves IV sodium bicarbonate (1–2 mEq/kg IV slowly over 20 min) to drive K^+ back into the cells. Slow intravenous administration of 0.5 U/kg of regular insulin coupled with 2 g of dextrose per unit of insulin can be also be administered. For refractory cases of hyperkalemia, calcium gluconate (0.5–1 mL of a 10% solution/kg) may be given by very slow intravenous administration, while monitoring the ECG.

AV block

In complete (third-degree) AV block, the ventricular escape rhythm is usually regular and below 40 bpm in dogs. In such cases, clinical signs such as lethargy or syncope are usually observed. If no underlying electrolyte abnormalities are present, a permanent pacemaker is the only effective treatment for this bradyarrhythmia. In cases with clinical signs due to second-degree AV block, medical management as described for sinus bradycardia can be attempted, but dogs might also require pacemaker implantation.

Complete AV block also occurs in cats, and is occasionally associated with hyperthyroidism. Cats with complete AVB can have "low-normal" HR due to a fast ventricular escape rhythm (120–140 bpm) and no overt clinical signs, but typically over time (months to years) the escape rate tends to diminish and once the HR drops below 100 bpm, cats start to show lethargy or syncope and may also develop congestive heart failure from chronic bradycardia. At that point, pacemaker therapy is indicated, just like in dogs. Due to cost, most cat owners elect medical therapy using beta agonists (Terbutaline), but the efficacy is very limited.

Treatment of ventricular arrhythmias (VAs)

The need for treatment of VA depends both on the hemodynamic consequences (i.e., hypotension causing weakness or fainting) and on the electrical instability of a rhythm (i.e., potential to degenerate into fatal ventricular fibrillation [VF]). Fainting or weakness is usually due to ventricular tachycardia (VT) rather than single or paired VPCs. Hypotension produced by VT is related to the heart rate and duration of VT and cardiac contractility. In most cases, sustained periods of VT >180–200 bpm are associated with clinical signs. The heart rate of VT is also linked to the electrical propensity to degenerate into VF, which is more likely in the setting of significant underlying heart disease.

Treatment may decrease clinical signs by slowing the heart rate of VT, shortening the duration of runs of VT, or, ideally, abolishing the VT entirely. However, no specific antiarrhythmic drug regimen has been shown to prevent sudden death due to VA. If systemic disease is present, it is important to correct electrolyte (K^+, Mg^{2+}) and acid–base disturbances, anemia, hypovolemia, or hypoxia, while managing the VA. Drugs commonly used for treatment of ventricular arrhythmias are presented in Table 4.3.

Treatment of acute, life-threatening VT

Dogs and cats with VT and severe systemic hypotension resulting in weakness or repeated collapsing require immediate IV treatment, with the goals of conversion to sinus rhythm or slowing of the VT rate. Intravenous treatment with a sodium-channel blocker, typically lidocaine, is the first choice for sustained VT. If lidocaine boluses are effective, a constant rate infusion (CRI) of lidocaine is started. Signs of lidocaine overdose include twitching, seizures, or vomiting, but side effects dissipate rapidly because of the drug's short half-life. Lidocaine is effective for VT in cats, but should be used judiciously due to the lower

threshold for seizures in cats. The antiarrhythmic effects of lidocaine are diminished in the presence of hypokalemia. Alternatives to lidocaine include procainamide given as a slow IV bolus, as it may cause vomiting or hypotension due its negative inotropic effect, followed by a CRI. Refractory VT may be treated with potassium-blocking antiarrhythmic agents, such as the IV form of water-soluble amiodarone-HCl (Nexterone). Nexterone is administered as an IV bolus infused over 10 min and is followed by a CRI. In cases of refractory VT, magnesium supplementation (30 mg/kg slowly IV) might also be beneficial.

Other agents such as BBs can be given for additive antiarrhythmic effect. Esmolol or propranolol IV boluses should be given judiciously because of the negative inotropic effect of BBs. Oral sotalol with or without simultaneous use of IV drugs can help convert dangerous VT to sinus rhythm within 1–3 hours. The negative inotropic effect of the BB component of sotalol should be considered.

Refractory VT, sometimes encountered in dogs with myocarditis, myocardial infarction, or myocardial neoplasia, might require electrical cardioversion, as was previously described for AF.

VF is not amenable to medical antiarrhythmic therapy, as organized cardiac electrical activity and function is absent, preventing delivery of peripherally injected drugs to the heart. Therefore, electric defibrillation is the treatment of choice for VF.

As previously mentioned, electrical cardioversion or defibrillation requires the patient to be anesthetized or unconscious. The animal is placed in dorsal or lateral recumbency and self-adhesive defibrillation pads or handheld defibrillation paddles are applied on opposites sides of the chest following application of conductive paste or gel. Different energy dosages are required, depending on whether the unit is a biphasic (0.5–3 J/kg) or monophasic defibrillator (2 J/kg: <7 kg BW; 5 J/kg: 8–40 kg BW; 5–10 J/kg: >40 kg BW). If the first shock is not effective, additional shocks of increasing energy are delivered.

Long-term therapy of VT

To determine whether an antiarrhythmic drug administered for long-term oral therapy of VA is having (1) an antiarrhythmic effect, (2) an inadequate effect, or (3) a proarrhythmic effect, Holter monitoring is recommended. A post-treatment Holter recording, acquired 7–10 days after starting the drug, is evaluated for changes in frequency or severity of the VA and to determine if treatment is having any proarrhythmic effects. The goal is to reduce clinical signs, such as frequency of syncope, and to eliminate or diminish runs of VT and number of VPCs by more than 85% compared with pre-treatment Holter. If the VA counts and severity are not sufficiently lowered, the drug dosage or regimen should be altered, and the Holter recording repeated 7–10 days later.

Sotalol is the most commonly prescribed oral antiarrhythmic for treatment of VA in dogs and cats because of its ability to reduce clinical signs and the low incidence of side effects. Dogs with severely decreased systolic function may need to be started on lower doses and titrated to effect, while monitoring for signs of low output or congestion. In dogs with VA associated with repolarization abnormalities or aggravated by bradycardia, such as German Shepherds with inherited ventricular arrhythmias and Boxers with bradycardia-associated syncope, sotalol is contraindicated as an initial sole treatment. In cases of refractory VT on sotalol, mexiletine, a sodium-channel blocker, can be combined with sotalol. The combination of mexiletine and atenolol is also an effective therapy for VT in Boxers with arrhythmogenic right ventricular cardiomyopathy (ARVC) and can be used if sotalol is deemed inadequate or proarrhythmic. Mexiletine can cause GI side effects (anorexia, vomiting, or diarrhea) and might also raise owner compliance issues, as it has to be given 3 times daily. In cats with occasional single VPCs and no clinical signs of collapse, atenolol monotherapy may be recommended.

For refractory VT, amiodarone is recommended, although its use is difficult because of the serious side effects reported in dogs (i.e., hepatoxicity, neutropenia, thyroid dysfunction). However, in dogs with life-threatening VT and poor contractility, it is a viable option as it does not affect contractility. Amiodarone can be combined with atenolol to enhance antiarrhythmic effects. Liver enzymes, complete blood cell counts, and thyroid function need to be monitored monthly for the first 3 months, and bimonthly thereafter. Propafenone is also used occasionally for refractory VT at 5–8 mg/kg 3 times daily, but its efficacy in dogs is considered anecdotal at this time. No published studies are available for use of amiodarone or propafenone in cats with arrhythmias.

REFERENCES

Meurs KM, Weidman JA, Rosenthal SL, Lahmers KK, Friedenberg SG. Ventricular arrhythmias in Rhodesian Ridgebacks with a family history of sudden death and results of a pedigree analysis for potential inheritance patterns. *J Am Vet Med Assoc* 2016, 248, 1135–1138.

Ware WA, Reina-Doreste Y, Stern JA, Meurs KM. Sudden death associated with QT interval prolongation and KCNQ1 gene mutation in a family of English Springer Spaniels. *J Vet Intern Med*. 2015, 29(2), 561–568. doi: 10.1111/jvim.12550. Epub 2015 Mar 16.

Section 5

HOLTER MONITORING

The diagnosis of intermittently occurring cardiac arrhythmias is challenging and typically requires ambulatory electrocardiography. Holter monitoring refers to ambulatory electrocardiogram (ECG) recording of the heart rate and rhythm over a prolonged period of time, ideally while the patient is in the familiar home environment and performs normal activities.

It is an important part of the diagnosis, screening, management, and prognosticating of arrhythmias. Even if a rhythm diagnosis is suspected based on the identification of occasional abnormal beats on an in-hospital ECG, a Holter monitor offers the best assessment of overall frequency and complexity of the arrhythmia and presents an important guide for monitoring treatment.

HOLTER INDICATIONS

- History of collapse or exercise intolerance—suspect sporadic arrhythmias
- Quantitation of arrhythmia burden of intermittent arrhythmias diagnosed by in-hospital ECGs
- Monitoring of drug efficacy—e.g., suppression of ventricular arrhythmias or ventricular rate control in atrial fibrillation
- Screening for arrhythmias in apparently healthy dogs of predisposed breeds at risk for cardiac disease

DEVICES AVAILABLE FOR CONTINUOUS AMBULATORY ECG MONITORING

The most commonly available device for short-term (24 h to 48 h) continuous monitoring is the Holter, worn externally with a vest (**Fig. 5.1**) for the duration of the recording, providing a three-lead ECG recording. It can be cumbersome for cat patients and of limited utility when longer-term monitoring is desirable (infrequent arrhythmias). Modern digital systems are quite small and light (**Figs. 5.2, 5.3, 5.5, and 5.6**) and secured on the animals back using specially designed vests or jackets, as well as adhesive bandages.

For infrequent arrhythmia capture, event monitors—also known as implantable loop recorders may be advantageous. They can continually record and overwrite a short section of a single-lead ECG trace. Subcutaneously implanted systems are smaller than a triple-A battery (**Fig. 5.4**) and capable of monitoring up to 3 years. Placed on the left hemithorax under

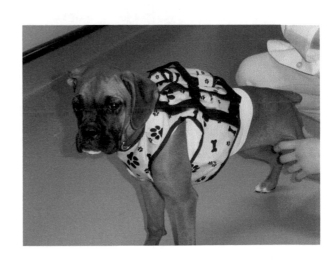

Fig. 5.1 Holter recorder, secured on dog with a specially designed vest where the monitor is carried in a pouch on the back.

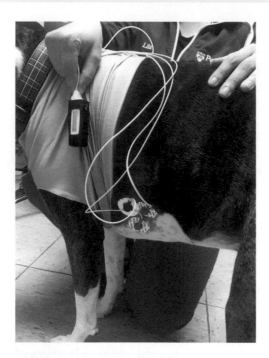

Fig. 5.2 The Holter system is secured with a dog shirt which has been folded forward to show the electrode positioning on the left hemithorax and the small monitor (Mortara Instruments) to be placed in a pouch on the dog's back. With this system, two additional electrodes are placed similarly on the right hemithorax.

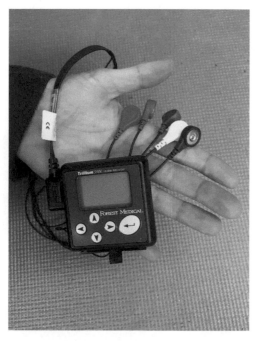

Fig. 5.3 Small digital Holter unit (Forest Medical, LLC) used for 24–48-hour recordings.

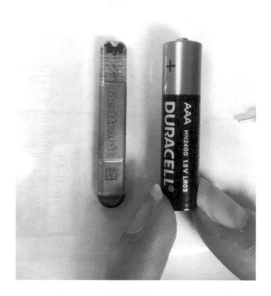

Fig. 5.4 Implantable loop recorder (LINQ, Medtronic), to be implanted under the skin on the left precordial impulse to monitor the ECG for up to 3 years.

sedation, they are well tolerated, but do not store the entire ECG recording; saving of episodes of interest is dependent on manual activation by the owner (i.e., after witnessing a collapse) or automatic activation.

Holter monitors differ from the loop recorders in that the ECG for the entire recording duration is stored and can be evaluated for abnormal beat counts, maximum, minimum, and average heart rate. Owners might be concerned that the recording may not be diagnostic if their pet does not show clinical signs, such as weakness or collapse, while wearing the monitor. Ideally, an ECG is recorded during a collapse episode, but useful information can still be gleaned from 24 to 48 hours of ECG data, even if the dog's arrhythmias do not result in clinical signs during the recording. Multi-lead recordings, accomplished by the application of three or more electrode patches, are less vulnerable to motion artefacts and may allow for improved detection of abnormal P waves and QRS complexes.

HOLTER MONITOR PLACEMENT
Skin preparation before applying the patch electrodes is critical to obtain a diagnostic ECG recording. Hair needs to be clipped using the shortest possible blade, and then the skin wiped with alcohol to remove oils and dried skin prior

to application of sticky electrodes. Sometimes the patch glue is reinforced with a few dabs of tissue glue to ensure electrodes remain in place for the duration of the recording. The required number of electrodes (varies from 3 to 7 between systems) are then attached. On very active dogs, a small 2*2-inch strip of elastic tape can also be applied over the electrodes on each side of the chest (Fig. 5.5) to keep electrodes and patches securely on the chest, before covering up the entire system and wires with a wearable vest or dog "shirt" (**Fig. 5.6**). Elasticated materials are generally more comfortable for the patients than adhesive bandage material.

Due to their small size, it is challenging to fit cats with Holter monitors and have them pursue their normal activity in the home environment, as recommended in dogs. This likely results in under-diagnosis and under-treatment of feline arrhythmias. Newer Holter systems are smaller and lighter, yet most cats are highly uncooperative when it comes to wearing any confining jacket required to carry even small monitors on their body. Even if tolerated, cats might restrict their activity, which likely diminishes the clinical value of the recording. As an alternative, Holter monitors can be placed on cats during a hospital overnight stay during which time the monitor might be placed alongside them in the cage; however, this also fails to record the ECG during normal activity in the home environment. For these reasons, Holter monitoring in cats is challenging and rarely performed.

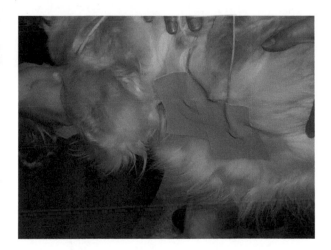

Fig. 5.5 Patch electrodes for a 24-hour Holter recording are placed on the dog's left hemithorax, after the hair has been clipped and the skin cleaned with alcohol. The electrodes are additionally taped to the dog's chest with a small strip of elasticon, before covering the system up with a vest or Surgi-Sox.

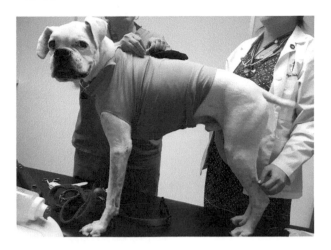

Fig. 5.6 Dog shirts ("Surgi-Sox" [DogLeggs, LLC]), modified by adding a small pouch to house the monitors, are very well tolerated by dogs as a Holter vest.

ANALYSIS OF HOLTER RECORDINGS

A variety of companies are available to perform Holter interpretation using proprietary commercial software to perform automated ECG analyses, aided by a manual review to ensure that artefacts are excluded and QRS complexes are accurately identified and correctly designated as being either narrow or wide QRS complexes to categorize as supraventricular or ventricular.

Typical Holter reports include the following information (**Fig. 5.7**):

- A total beat count (number of QRS complexes over entire recording): The total beat count per minute (mean heart rate during each minute of the recording) may be graphically displayed against time to provide a rate histogram (**Fig. 5.8**). This allows for interpretation of heart rate trends over the recording period that can be associated with dog activity (i.e., travel to and from the vet office, exercise, sleep vs. wake periods, etc.).
- Mean heart rate (average heart rate over the entire 24–48-hour period): In dogs, the 24-hour mean heart rate is typically in the range of 65–85 bpm. Maximum heart rate and minimum heart rate are usually provided based on short periods, ranging from an 8-second to a 1-minute average. *Table 5.1* provides normal heart rates derived from Holter recordings in dogs. The mean difference in heart rate between dogs weighing 5 and 55 kg is only 10.5 bpm and unlikely to be clinically significant.
- Abnormal beat counts summarizing ventricular arrhythmias and supraventricular arrhythmias:

Beat Counts

Normal Beats	VE Beats	SVE Beats	Paced Beats
Count **214,331**	Count **21,684**	Count **0**	Count **0**
Percent **91 %**	Percent **9 %**	Percent **0%**	Percent **0%**
Max/Hr **9,721** on Fri 17:00	Max/Hr **1,829** on Sat 01:00	Max/Hr **0** on	Max/Hr **0** on

Rate Dependent Events

Heart Rates (1 min avg)		Bradycardia **0**		Tachycardia	**17,303**
Max HR	**194 bpm** on Fri 17:12	Total		Total	**11 hr 6 min 45 sec, 46.4%**
Mean HR	**167 bpm**	Longest		Longest	**53 beats** on Sat 03:26
Min HR	**128 bpm** on Sat 06:13	Min Rate		Max Rate	**284 bpm** on Fri 17:08
Pause	0				

Ventricular Arrhythmias / Supraventricular Arrhythmias

Ventricular Arrhythmias		Supraventricular Arrhythmias	
VT	**2**, 0.0% of total beats (0 per 1000)	**AF**	**1 episodes**
Longest	**11 beats** on Sat 05:48	Total Duration	**23 hr 56 min 58 sec, 100.0%**
Max Rate	**233 bpm** on Sat 03:30	Max Rate	**287 bpm** on Fri 16:09
V-Run	**0**, 0.0% of total beats (0 per 1000)	**SVT**	**0**
Longest		Longest	
Max Rate		Max Rate	
Couplet	**65**, 0.1% of total beats (0 per 1000)	**SVE**	**0**, 0.0% of total beats (0 per 1000)
Triplet	**1**, 0.0% of total beats (0 per 1000)		
Single VE Events	**17,903**, 7.6% of total beats (76 per 1000)		

Indications (reason for test) :

Test Comments :

Findings :

The recording showed atrial fibrillation and very frequent ventricular ectopy (VE) that occurred as single beats and as more complex ectopy, including 1 short episode of ventricular tachycardia and 1 of accelerated idioventricular rhythm (both labelled by the software as ventricular tachycardia). The mean 24h heart rate was 167bpm.

During the reported episode of collapse (between 14.45-14.55) the rhythm was atrial fibrillation (heart rate between 165-180bpm) with presence of ventricular premature complexes that occurred mainly as single beats.

Fig. 5.7 Sample 24-hour Holter report in a dog with atrial fibrillation and ventricular arrhythmias.

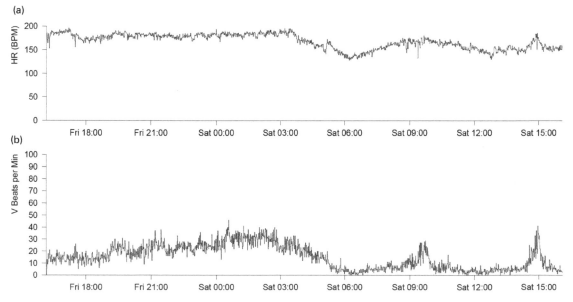

Fig. 5.8 Rate histogram (a) and ventricular beat frequency (b) over the course of the 24-hour recording: Time is on the horizontal axis (24-hour clock) and 1-minute average heart rates (bpm) (a), as well as frequency of ventricular beats per minute (b), on the vertical axes.

Ventricular arrhythmias are identified by a wide-complex QRS, while supraventricular beats are defined by their degree of prematurity. Manual review of automated analyses is needed to identify wide complex QRS complexes during sinus rhythm due to abnormal ventricular conduction (i.e., bundle branch block). The Holter report should provide a total abnormal beat count and quantify whether or not there is complex ventricular ectopy (such as couplets, triplets, or ventricular tachycardia), as well as the maximum number of consecutive ventricular beats and maximum heart rate of the tachycardia episodes. Occasional ventricular escape beats during periods of low heart rate are a normal finding in dogs. Up to 50 single ventricular premature beats/24 h can occur in normal dogs other than Boxers. However, even if the total number of ventricular premature beats is within normal limits, presence of complex ventricular ectopy such as couplets, triplets, or ventricular tachycardia is abnormal. Significant day-to-day variation in the frequency and complexity of ventricular ectopy occurs in dogs, which is why longer recording periods (i.e., 7-day or loop recorders) are sometimes indicated. Normal Holter findings in dogs based on previous studies are listed in *Tables 5.1* and *5.2*.

Table 5.1 Normal 24-hour Holter ECG findings in dogs

Parameters	24-hour Holter ECG findings
Heart rhythm	Sinus and sinus arrhythmia
Mean 24-hour heart rate (HR)	66 (52–86) bpm
Minimum 24-hour HR	38 (29–52) bpm
Maximum 24-hour HR	171 (130–240) bpm; during periods of intense exercise/excitement sinus tachycardia may briefly reach instantaneous rates >300 bpm
Sinus pauses	4–6 seconds at rest
Escape beats	Occasional during low heart rates
2nd AVB	Rare during periods of low heart rate
Ventricular premature beats	Uncommon, 0–91 (see Table 5.2)

Abbreviation: AVB, atrioventricular block

Table 5.2 Ventricular premature beat counts in normal dogs

Breed	VPCs/24 h
Beagles	<9
Large breed dogs	0–24
Boxers	<91
Doberman Pinschers	<50
Salukis	0–4

ANTIARRHYTHMIC TREATMENT ASSESSMENT UTILIZING 24-HOUR HOLTER DATA

Ideally, antiarrhythmic therapy efficacy should be assessed by comparing a pre-treatment and post-treatment (1–2 weeks after initiating medical therapy) Holter recording. In cases where ventricular tachycardia is observed on in-hospital ECGs or very frequent fainting, a pre-treatment Holter may not be acquired so as to avoid delay in the initiation of therapy. However, the absence of pre-treatment Holter data makes it difficult to fully assess the response to therapy. Comparing pre-treatment and post-treatment Holter recordings might also reveal potential proarrhythmic drug effects and allow evaluation of treatment efficacy. Because of considerable day-to-day variability in VPC number, an adequate treatment response should yield at least an 80% reduction in VPC number and a reduction in the complexity of the arrhythmia on the post-treatment Holter.

Specifically, identification of frequent ventricular ectopy in an adult Boxer or Doberman Pinscher is strongly suggestive of a diagnosis of arrhythmogenic right ventricular cardiomyopathy (ARVC) or dilated cardiomyopathy, respectively, particularly if there is significant complexity (couplets, triplets, bigeminy, or ventricular tachycardia) in the absence of other underlying systemic or cardiac disease that could cause ventricular arrhythmias.

Rate control for dogs with chronic atrial fibrillation is also best assessed using 24-hour Holter recordings in the home environment, as in-hospital ECGs tend to overestimate the ventricular rate of dogs with atrial fibrillation. Sympathetic stimulation from the stress of being in a hospital setting and dog handling for ECG acquisition produce markedly elevated heart rates as compared to 24-hour-average heart rates recorded by Holter in a familiar setting, making in-hospital ECGs of limited value for interpretation of drug efficacy in this arrhythmia.

ECG CASES

Question 1

ECG recorded from an 11-year-old Golden Retriever with acute onset of extreme weakness.

1 What are the findings in **ECG 1** (50 mm/s; 10 mm/mV)?
2 What is the clinical significance of this ECG?

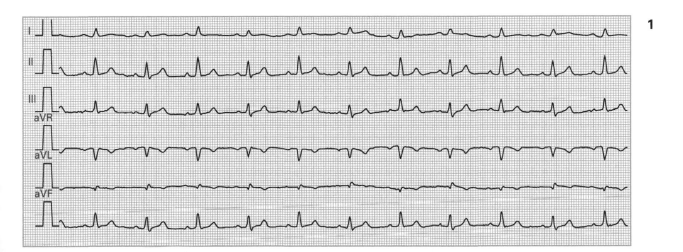

1

Question 2

Lead II ECG recorded in a 3-year-old Labrador Retriever.

1 What are the findings in **ECG 2** (25 mm/s; 20 mm/mV)?
2 What is the clinical significance of this ECG?

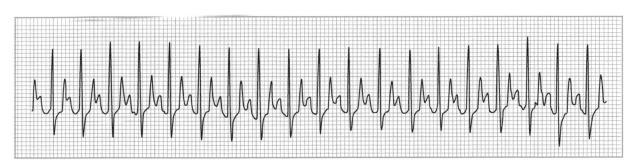

2

Answer 1

1 ECG 1 shows sinus rhythm with low amplitude QRS complexes and electrical alternans.

2 • The heart rate is ~145 bpm. The P wave amplitude is normal. The QRS amplitude in all leads is <1.0 mV which is unusual for a large breed dog. The R wave height varies slightly with every other beat, most easily appreciated in leads II and aVF. Beat to beat variation in QRS complex amplitude or configuration is called electrical alternans.

• Low amplitude QRS complexes and electrical alternans are most commonly found in association with pericardial effusion. These findings are not extremely sensitive, but fairly specific for pericardial effusion. Dampening of the electrical signal by the pericardial effusion decreases the QRS amplitude, and swinging of the heart in the fluid-filled pericardial sac is considered the origin of the electrical alternans.

• Large volumes of pericardial effusion impair cardiac filling, resulting in cardiogenic shock (pericardial tamponade), and require pericardiocentesis and often intravenous fluid administration. In this patient, pericardial effusion was confirmed by echocardiography and a mass was visualized originating at the right atrium. The right atrial mass is most likely a hemangiosarcoma, which is commonly diagnosed in older, large breed dogs with pericardial effusion.

Answer 2

1 ECG 2 shows either SVT or sinus tachycardia.

2 • The average heart rate is 200 bpm. The rhythm is regular.

• There is a P wave (blue arrow), QRS complex (black arrow), and T wave (green arrow) for every beat.

• The rapid heart rate causes the P wave to be partially obscured by the preceding T wave.

• The QRS complex morphology is normal indicating a supraventricular origin, which could be ectopic (SVT) or originating from the sinus node (sinus tachycardia).

• Differentiation between the two rhythms can sometimes be difficult. SVT is characterized by sudden (paroxysmal) stopping and starting of the tachycardia, electrical alternans (cyclical variation in the amplitude of the QRS complex), changes in P wave morphology, persistence despite sedation or alleviation of patient stress, and underlying myocardial or valvular disease. In contrast, sinus tachycardia is usually associated with gradual acceleration and deceleration of the tachycardia, disappearance when patient stress is alleviated, and normal underlying heart function.

• Labrador Retrievers are particularly prone to SVT and may require additional diagnostic procedures, such as echocardiography or 24-hour ambulatory (Holter) monitoring, as well as medical therapy to slow the heart rate (i.e., beta-blockers, calcium-channel blockers, digoxin).

2
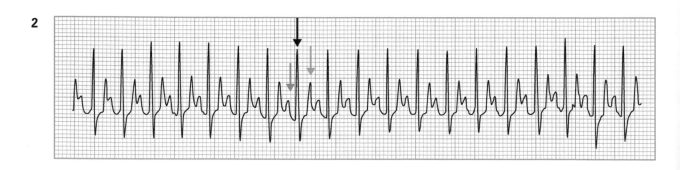

Question 3

ECG recorded in a 5-year-old Great Dane dog.

1 What are the findings in **ECG 3** (50 mm/s; 10 mm/mV)?
2 What is the clinical significance of this ECG?

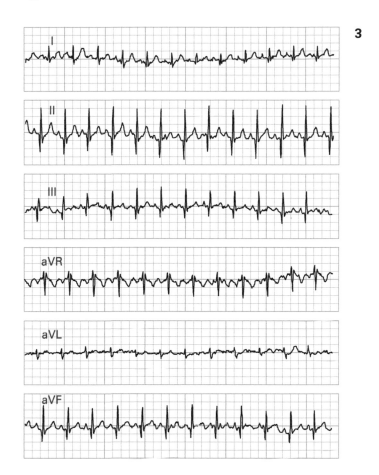

Question 4

ECG recorded from a 9-year-old male mixed breed dog that presents to the emergency service with acute collapse.

1 What are the findings in **ECG 4** (50 mm/s; 10 mm/mV)?
2 What is the clinical significance of this ECG?

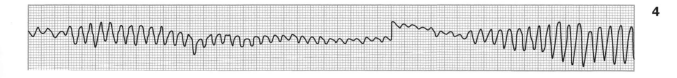

Answer 3

1 ECG 3 shows sinus tachycardia.
2 • The average heart rate is 200 bpm and the rhythm is regular. There is a normal P, QRS, and
   T wave for each beat.
  • Sinus tachycardia is mediated by increased sympathetic tone and can be a normal response to stress
    or exercise, or secondary to systemic conditions such as sepsis, fever, hypovolemia, shock, or heart
    failure.
  • Sinus tachycardia can be differentiated from SVT through its gradual acceleration and deceleration in
    response to stress and the absence of other clinical signs in instances of excitement or exercise.

Answer 4

1 ECG 4 demonstrates a particular type of polymorphic VT called torsade de pointes.
2 • There is a characteristic illusion of a twisting of the QRS complex around the baseline. The ECG has
   an undulating appearance with varying QRS amplitudes. Torsade de pointes can degenerate into VF,
   which is a terminal arrhythmia if not quickly defibrillated.
  • Various causes have been implicated in this dangerous arrhythmia, including adverse effects from
    certain sodium- or potassium-channel blocking antiarrhythmic drugs, and/or electrolyte or metabolic
    disturbances (hypokalemia, hypocalcemia, hypomagnesemia, acidosis) that prolong the QT interval.
    VPCs in the presence of long QT intervals predispose the patient to an R-on-T phenomenon,
    where the R wave of a subsequent beat occurs during the relative refractory period at the end of
    repolarization (T wave) of the preceding beat, and thus may initiate torsades or fibrillation.
  • For this arrhythmia, treatment is directed at withdrawal of the offending agent, infusion of
    magnesium sulfate, and/or electrical defibrillation.

Question 5

ECG recorded from a 5-year-old Newfoundland dog with an arrhythmia.

1 What are the findings in **ECG 5** (25 mm/s; 10 mm/mV)?
2 What is the clinical significance of this ECG?

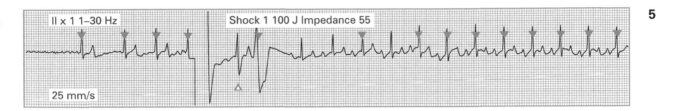

Question 6

ECG recorded in a 12-year-old male castrated Golden Retriever with a heart murmur.

1 What are the findings in **ECG 6** (25 mm/s; 5 mm/mV)?
2 What is the clinical significance of this ECG?

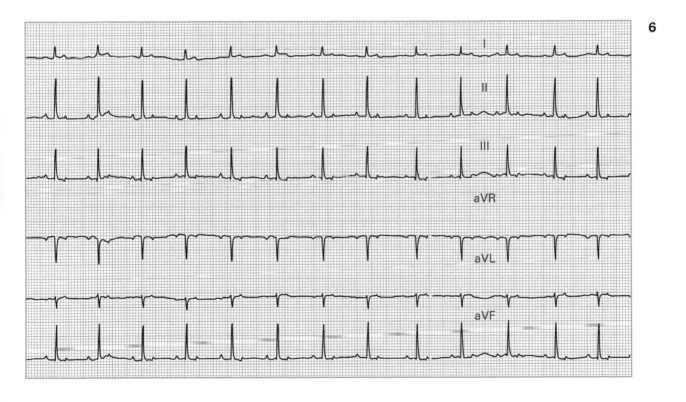

Answer 5

1 **ECG 5** shows conversion to sinus rhythm, using electrical cardioversion.

2 • The initial four complexes represent AF, with a ventricular rate of approximately 60 bpm. AF is diagnosed based on the absence of distinct P waves, presence of low amplitude f waves, the irregular nature of the rhythm, and the QRS complexes having supraventricular morphology (see **ECG 12**, p. 59 and **ECG 29**, p. 81).

• Because of the absence of significant underlying heart disease and the relatively slow ventricular rate, a diagnosis of "lone" AF was made and conversion back to sinus rhythm was attempted using electrical cardioversion. A transthoracic electrical shock was delivered with a biphasic defibrillator (blue and white arrowheads).

• The small blue arrows pointing to the R waves are synchronization markers. Defibrillation shocks should never be delivered over the T wave, since the repolarization phase is a vulnerable window for induction of VF. To avoid this complication, the defibrillator detects the R waves and synchronizes the defibrillation discharge with the onset of the R wave.

• Immediately following cardioversion, there are two ventricular beats (red arrows), followed by restoration of sinus rhythm with normal P waves (purple arrows) and QRS complexes (green arrow).

5

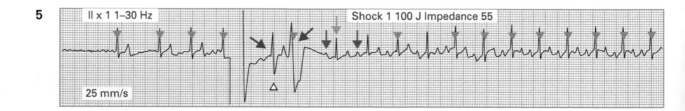

Answer 6

1 **ECG 6** shows sinus rhythm.

2 • The heart rate is ~94 bpm. The rhythm is regular and there is a P for every QRS and QRS for every P. The amplitude and duration of the P and QRS complexes are normal. The QRS complex amplitude is 2.6 mV. In order for the QRS complexes from each lead to fit onto the paper without overlapping each other, note that the ECG sensitivity was set at 5 mm/mV, which is half the normal (10 mm/mV) setting. The MEA is normal.

• Sinus rhythm represents the normal sequence of cardiac depolarization. In the dog, sinus rhythm typically ranges between 70 and 180 bpm, although in large breed dogs, the upper rate is often defined as 140 bpm, and in puppies, 220 bpm.

• The key points are the regularity, and normal rate, sequence, and morphology of the P–QRS–T waves.

Question 7

ECG recorded in a 9-year-old male domestic shorthair cat with a grade 2/6 systolic murmur.

1 What are the findings in **ECG 7** (50 mm/s; 10 mm/mV)?
2 What is the clinical significance of this ECG?

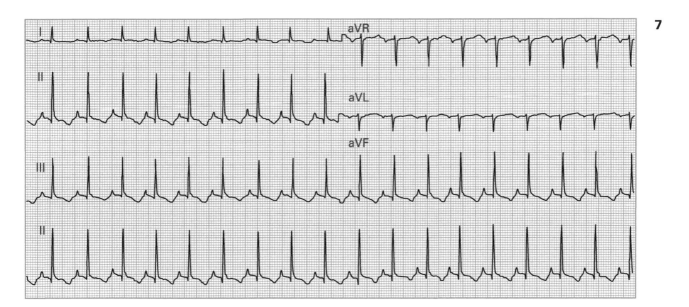

7

Question 8

ECG from a 9-year-old Collie being treated for glomerulonephritis and progressive respiratory distress and tachycardia.

1 What are the findings in **ECG 8** (50 mm/s; 10 mm/mV)?
2 What is the clinical significance of this ECG?

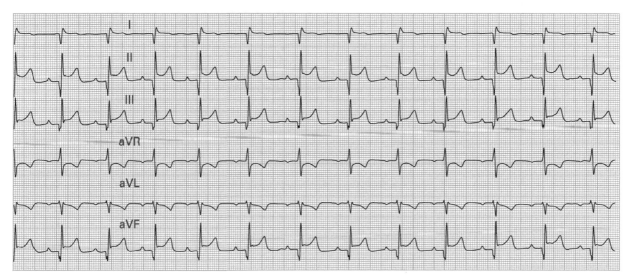

8

Answer 7

1 ECG 7 shows sinus rhythm with evidence of left ventricular hypertrophy.

2 • The average heart rate is 210 bpm. The rhythm is regular.
  • The amplitude of the R wave in lead II is 1.9 mV (normal <0.9 mV) suggesting left ventricular hypertrophy. The caudal limb leads III and aVF, which are similar in orientation to lead II, also display R wave amplitudes similar to lead II.
  • Left ventricular enlargement is often due to cardiomyopathy or, less commonly, hyperthyroidism or systemic hypertension. Based on the ECG findings as well as the presence of a heart murmur, underlying changes in cardiac structure and function are likely, and further diagnostics, such as radiographs or echocardiography, are warranted.

Answer 8

1 ECG 8 shows sinus rhythm with ST segment elevation.

2 • The heart rate is 150 bpm. The ST segment is markedly elevated (arrows) in leads II, III, and aVF and depressed in lead aVR. The Q waves are notched in leads II, III, and aVF.
  • ST segment elevation or depression occurs secondary to myocardial hypoxia/ischemia in dogs and cats. In humans, the discrete location of a recent myocardial infarction can often be inferred based on ST segment changes. The mechanisms underlying ST segment changes are complex. Hypoxic conditions in the myocardium leads to diminished intracellular concentrations of adenosine triphosphate (ATP), and thus decreased activity of ATP-dependent ion transport systems. These systems play an important role in maintenance of the resting cell membrane as well as action potential propagation. In cases of myocardial hypoxemia, neighboring regions of myocardium will have different electrical properties and a small electrical current (current of injury) flows from the depolarized ischemic regions to more normal regions, resulting in ST segment elevation or depression.
  • In this case, pulmonary thromboembolism secondary to glomerulonephritis and loss of antithrombin III resulted in severe hypoxemia.

8

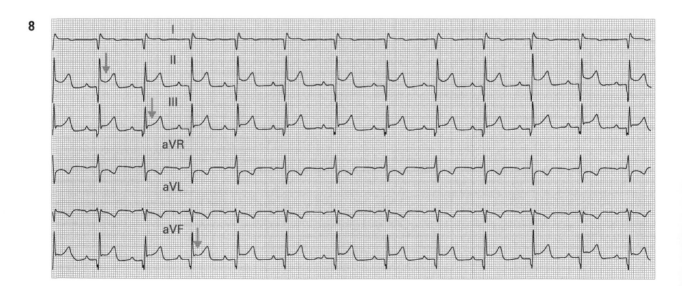

Question 9

ECG recorded from an 8-year-old Lhasa Apso presented for yearly vaccinations, and an arrhythmia was ausculted.

1 What are the findings in **ECG 9** (50 mm/s; 10 mm/mV)?
2 What is the clinical significance of this ECG?

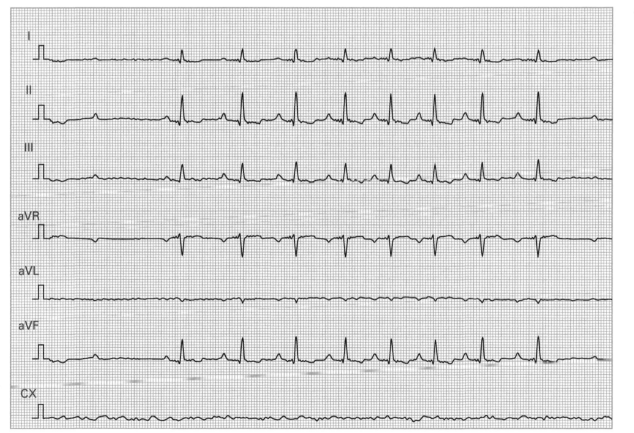

Answer 9

1 ECG 9 shows second-degree AV nodal block.
2 • There are P waves that are not followed by a QRS (arrowheads). This is an example of Mobitz type I (Wenckebach) AV block, wherein the PR interval gradually prolongs before a P wave is blocked. The arrows displaying the PR interval are longer at the end of the sequence of sinus beats than at the beginning.
  • Second-degree AV block can be due to high-resting vagal tone, degeneration or infiltration of the AV node, or infectious or inflammatory disease. In patients with high vagal tone and slow heart rates, Wenckebach type second-degree AV block can occasionally be observed as a physiological phenomenon. In this case, the underlying heart rate is relatively high at 150 bpm, indicating that vagal tone is not predominant and underlying disease of the AV node is likely. In cases of infrequent AV block, no clinical signs are observed and no treatment is indicated. In cases of frequent AV block and resulting bradycardia, syncope or weakness can result.
  • Atropine (0.04 mg/kg) can be administered intravenously or subcutaneously in an attempt to resolve the AV block. Incomplete resolution of the AV block suggests presence of underlying AV nodal injury or disease.

9

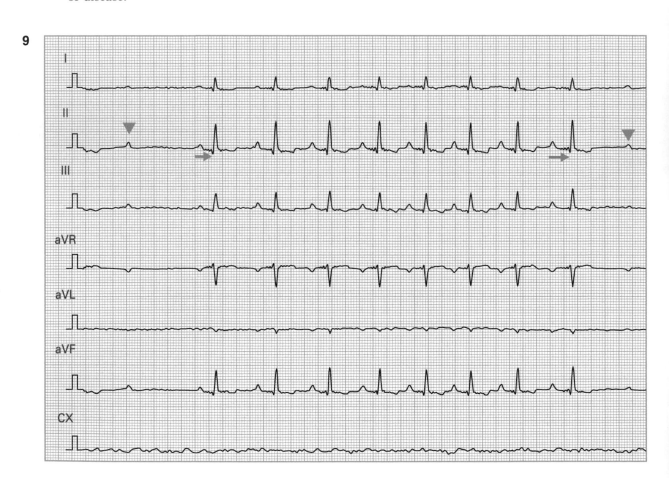

Question 10
ECG recorded in a 9-year-old male castrated Cocker Spaniel with a heart murmur.

1 What are the findings in **ECG 10** (25 mm/s; 10 mm/mV)?
2 What is the clinical significance of this ECG?

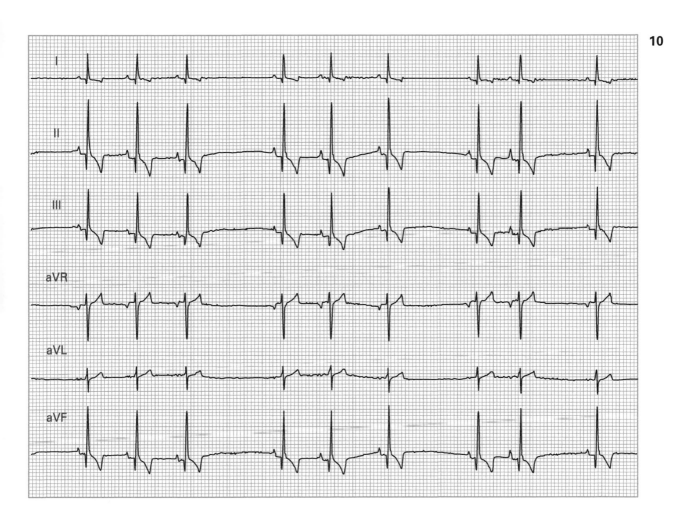

Answer 10

1 **ECG 10** shows sinus arrhythmia.
2 • The average heart rate is ~90 bpm. The rhythm is regularly irregular and there is a P for every QRS and QRS for every P. The amplitude and duration of the P and QRS complexes are normal. The MEA is normal.
   • Sinus arrhythmia is similar to sinus rhythm with respect to average heart rate and the normal sequence of cardiac depolarization. Sinus arrhythmia differs from sinus rhythm in that the heart rate demonstrates phasic changes that are often (but not always) related to respiration. Higher rates are noted during inspiration and slower heart rates during expiration (respiratory sinus arrhythmia).
   • Changes in size and shape of the P wave (arrows) is termed wandering pacemaker and can occur during sinus arrhythmia. The P wave amplitude is greater during faster heart rates and smaller during slower heart rates.
   • Vagolytic stimuli (e.g., exercise, atropine) reduces or eliminates sinus arrhythmia.
   • The key points are the phasic irregularity and normal rate, sequence, and morphology of the P–QRS–T waves.

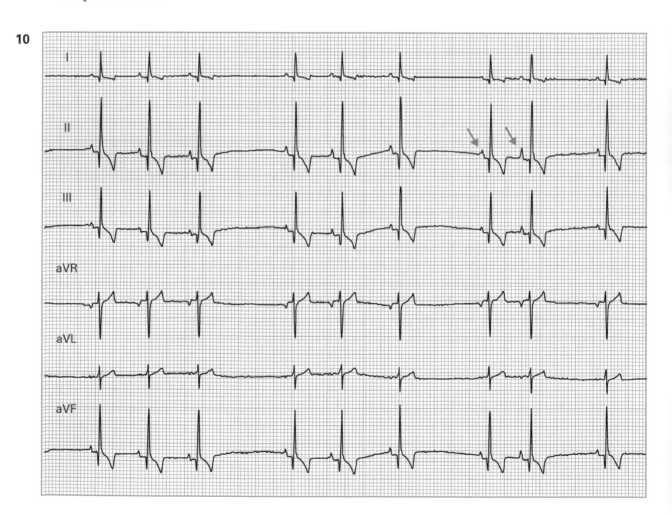

Question 11

ECG recorded from a 5-year-old Siberian Husky.

1 What are the findings in **ECG 11** (25 mm/s; 10 mm/mV)?
2 What is the clinical significance of this ECG?

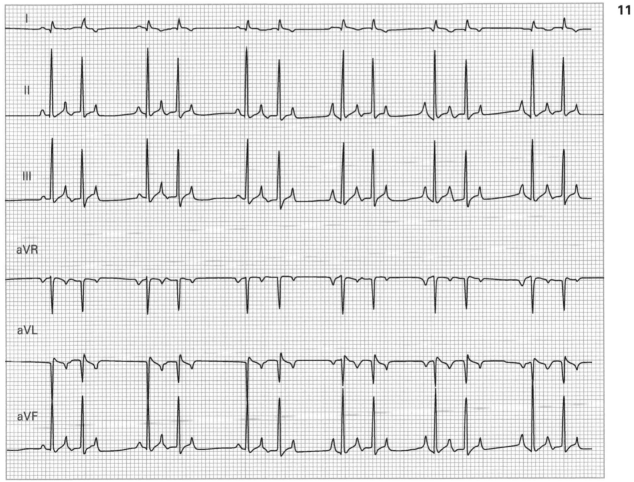

11

Answer 11

1 ECG 11 shows atrial premature complexes.

2 • The average heart rate is 135 bpm. The rhythm is regularly irregular with beats occurring in pairs. The first beat is a sinus beat and the second beat is an atrial premature beat. There is a normal P wave in front of the sinus QRS complex of each pair. The atrial premature beat has a normal QRS configuration and a small negative P wave (arrows).

• The interval between the first and second beat of each pair equates to an atrial premature beat rate of 190 bpm. The term *atrial bigeminy* is often used in instances when the sinus and atrial premature beats alternate in a regular 1:1 fashion.

• Atrial premature beats often occur in cases with underlying heart diseases, especially in those that produce atrial enlargement (i.e., mitral valve disease, cardiomyopathy), but can also be secondary to a wide variety of extracardiac conditions.

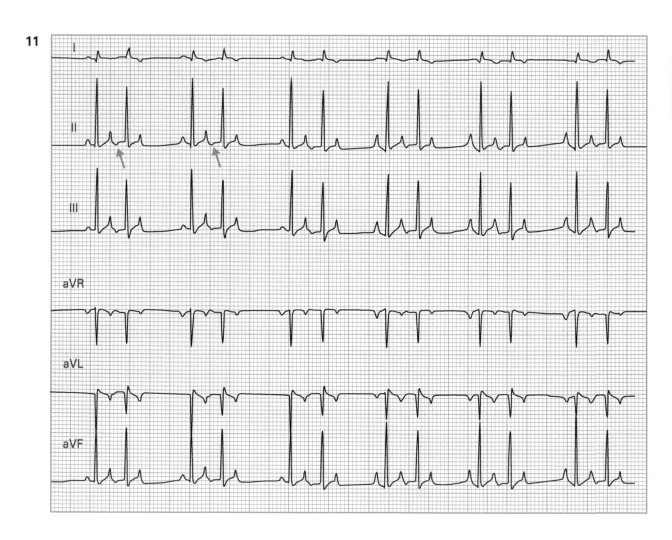

Question 12
ECG recorded in an 8-year-old male castrated domestic shorthair cat.

1 What are the findings in **ECG 12** (50 mm/s; 10 mm/mV)?
2 What is the clinical significance of this ECG?

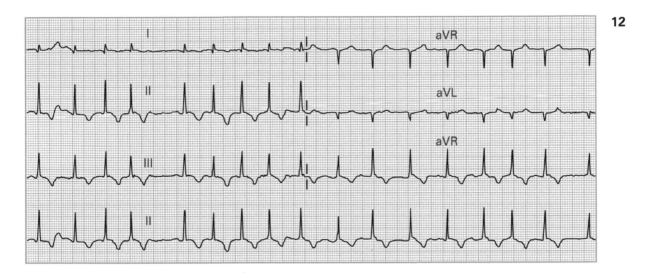

Question 13
ECG recorded from a 6-year-old Boxer that presented with a 3-week history of progressive coughing and onset of severe dyspnea over the last 48 hours.

1 What are the findings in **ECG 13** (50 mm/s; 10 mm/mV)?
2 What is the clinical significance of this ECG?

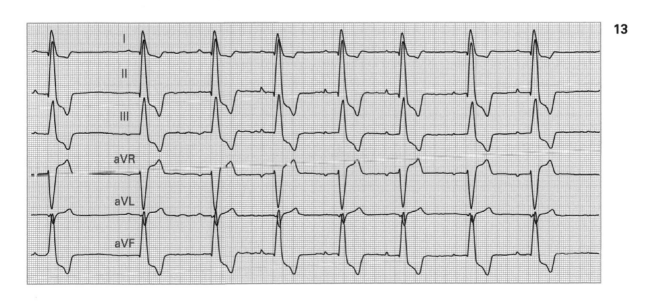

Answer 12

1 **ECG 12** shows atrial fibrillation (AF) and left ventricular enlargement.
2 • The heart rate ranges from 130 bpm to 272 bpm, with the average ~220 bpm. The rhythm is irregularly irregular.
   • There are no consistent P waves noted; however, despite the lack of P waves, the QRS complexes are narrow and appear to be of supraventricular origin.
   • The amplitude is 1.3 mV (normal <0.9 mV) indicating left ventricular enlargement. Note that the caudal limb leads III and aVF, which are similar in orientation with lead II, also display QRS complex amplitudes that are relatively increased, further supporting left ventricular enlargement.
   • The irregularity, lack of P waves, and supraventricular QRS complexes are all findings consistent with AF.
   • In cats, AF is usually due to severe underlying heart disease, and further diagnostics such as radiographs and echocardiography are indicated.
   • Treatment of AF involves slowing the ventricular rate by decreasing conduction through the AV node with medications such as beta-blockers, calcium-channel blockers, and/or digoxin.

Answer 13

1 **ECG 13** shows sinus rhythm with a left bundle branch block (LBBB).
2 • The heart rate is 100 bpm. The QRS complexes look wide and bizarre, and the duration is prolonged at 100 ms. The MEA is normal. The rhythm is sinus in origin as evidenced by the fact that there are P waves preceding each QRS complex, with a regular PR interval of 140 ms. The P wave morphology changes slightly with heart rate, indicating a wandering pacemaker. The PR interval is slightly prolonged, consistent with first-degree AV block. The ST segment is depressed and slurred, which is suggestive of myocardial hypoxia.
   • The diagnosis of a LBBB is made based on sinus QRS complexes with a normal MEA and increased duration of the QRS (>80 ms in a dog, >50 ms in a cat). The wide QRS duration is caused by complete disruption of the left bundle branch and delayed depolarization of the left ventricle.
   • The QRS complex morphology of LBBB mimics that of a VPC. The key feature discriminating between LBBB and VPCs is the presence of P waves associated with each QRS, signifying the QRS as supraventricular in origin. If the heart rate is very rapid, the P waves may be hidden in the preceding T waves, and the rhythm can be difficult to discern from VT.
   • LBBB almost never occurs by itself as a benign abnormality. Rather, it occurs secondary to left ventricular myocardial disease (cardiomyopathy, mitral valve disease) or degenerative conduction system disease. While the LBBB does not require treatment per se, the presence of underlying cardiac disease results in a relatively poor prognosis. The finding of LBBB should prompt further diagnostics such as echocardiography to search for an underlying cardiac disease.

Question 14
A 10-year-old cat presented for a dental prophylaxis.

1 What are the findings in **ECG 14** (50 mm/s, 10 mm/mV)?
2 What is the clinical significance of this ECG?

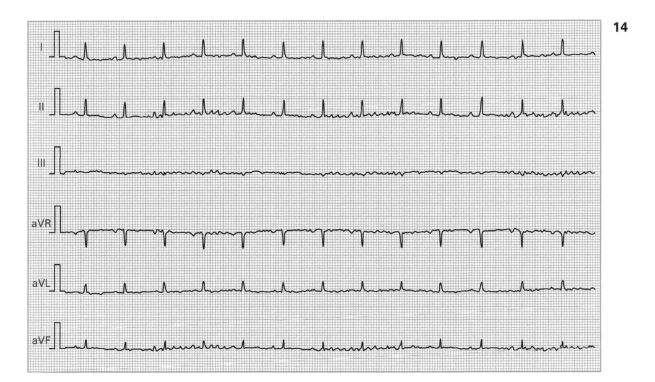

14

Question 15
ECG recorded from an 8-year-old Rottweiler that presents for several episodes of collapse.

1 What are the findings in **ECG 15** (50 mm/s; 10mm/mV)?
2 What is the clinical significance of this ECG?

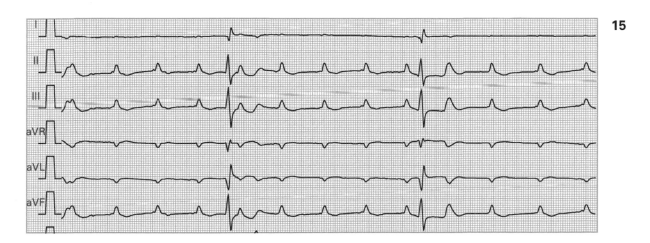

15

Answer 14

1 ECG 14 shows normal sinus rhythm with baseline artifact.
2 • The heart rate is 200 bpm, likely in response to being handled for ECG acquisition. The P–QRS–T complexes are normal and the MEA is normal.
  • The diastolic intervals after the third and fourth QRS complex, the sixth and eighth, as well as the eleventh and twelfth QRS complexes show small, high-frequency undulations, most easily discerned in leads II and aVF. These undulations are not an arrhythmia, but the consequence of the cat purring, causing a repeatable, breathing-associated artifact in this ECG. This type of artifact can often be mistaken as AF, but the presence of P waves precludes this diagnosis. In dogs, panting or shivering are common causes of similar artifacts. Other causes of ECG artifact include electrical current 60 or 50 Hz interference, due to poor grounding of the ECG machine or any other electronic equipment connected to the patient. The 60 Hz cycle interference can also mimic AF, and all other electronic equipment in the room may need to be unplugged to avoid this artifact.

Answer 15

1 ECG 15 shows complete or third-degree AV nodal block.
2 • The ventricular heart rate is 35 bpm. There is complete AV dissociation, with the P waves having no relationship to the QRS complexes and the atrial and ventricular rates are independent of each other. In complete AV block, the atrial rate (P–P interval) is always faster than the ventricular rate, and P waves should have ample opportunity to conduct to the ventricles, but fail to do so. In third-degree (complete) AV block, the ventricular escape rhythm is usually slow and regular, and approximately 40–60 bpm in dogs and 80–120 bpm in cats.
  • The etiology of most cases of third-degree AV block is unknown, but age-related degeneration of the AV node or acute myocarditis are two possible causes.
  • Most dogs with third-degree AV block show signs of weakness, lethargy, activity intolerance, or syncope, and require artificial pacemaker implantation. In cats, the more rapid ventricular escape rate often permits normal quality of life without the need for any specific therapy.

Question 16

ECG recorded in an 11-year-old mixed breed dog.

1 What are the findings in **ECG 16** (25 mm/s; 10 mm/mV)?
2 What is the clinical significance of this ECG?

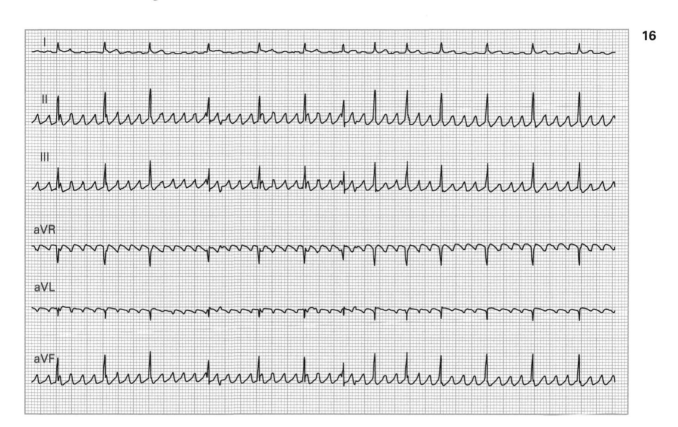

16

Question 17

ECG recorded in a domestic shorthair cat.

1 What are the findings in **ECG 17** (25 mm/s; 10 mm/mV)?
2 What is the clinical significance of this ECG?

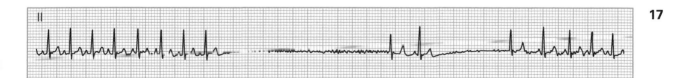

17

Answer 16

1 ECG 16 shows atrial flutter (AFL).
2 • The average heart rate is 120 bpm. The rhythm is irregular and there is a "sawtooth" baseline that represents the AFL waves (F waves). The rate of the F waves is 425 bpm. The QRS complexes are narrow and of normal morphology.
 • AFL usually occurs in the presence of advanced cardiac disease, such as mitral valve disease or dilated cardiomyopathy. AFL is often considered a more "organized" form of AF. The ventricular rate is dependent on the conduction of the F waves through the AV node and is further described by the ratio of F waves to QRS complexes (e.g., four F waves for every one QRS is described as 4:1). In cases where the ventricular rate is rapid, medication to slow conduction through the AV node (e.g., digoxin, diltiazem, and/or atenolol) can be used.
 • The key points are the "sawtooth baseline" made up of F waves, the variable conduction of F waves through the AV node, and the often rapid ventricular rate.

Answer 17

1 ECG 17 shows sinus arrest and junctional escape beats.
2 • There are eight beats of sinus rhythm at the start of the ECG tracing with normal P waves, QRS complexes, and T waves. The heart rate is ~215 bpm and the rhythm is regular.
 • Following the eighth beat, there is a 2.5-second period of sinus arrest that is terminated by a narrow QRS complex without a P wave, consistent with a junctional escape beat. This is followed by another sinus beat, a second period of sinus arrest, a second junctional escape beat, and then resumption of sinus rhythm. Sinus arrest can be secondary to sinus node disease, cardiomyopathy, abnormal vagal tone secondary to central nervous system, gastrointestinal, or respiratory disease, or drug toxicity (i.e., beta-blockers). Extended periods of sinus arrest (typically >3–4 seconds in cats) can cause clinical signs such as syncope or weakness.

Question 18

ECG recorded from a 15-year-old domestic shorthair cat admitted for a dental examination with a grade 2/6 systolic heart murmur.

1 What are the findings in **ECG 18** (50 mm/s; 10 mm/mV)?
2 What is the clinical significance of this ECG?

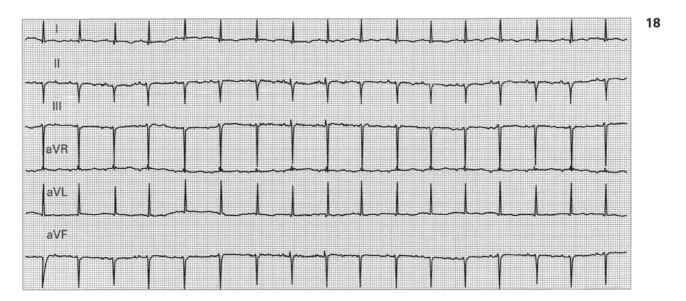

18

Question 19

ECG recorded from a 6-year-old male castrated Boxer that presents for collapse during exercise.

1 What are the findings in **ECG 19** (50 mm/s; 10 mm/mV)?
2 What is the clinical significance of this ECG?

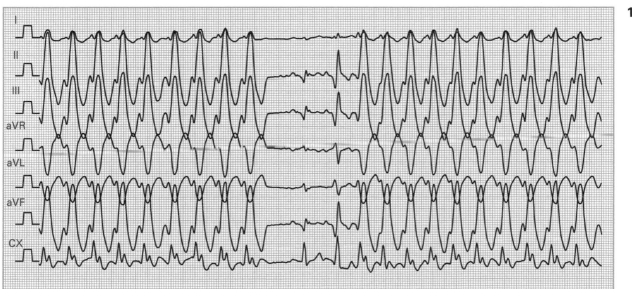

19

Answer 18

1 ECG 18 shows sinus rhythm with a left anterior fascicular block (LAFB) pattern.
2 • The heart rate is 200 bpm. The MEA is shifted to the left to –50° (see Section 2, Evaluation of the Electrocardiogram). The QRS duration is 20 ms and normal.
  • The LAFB pattern is thought to arise from disruption of the anterior fascicule of the left bundle branch that supplies the cranial and basilar region of the left ventricle with electrical impulses. A region of block will result in a deviation of the MEA of the ventricular depolarization to the left, but the QRS duration is not prolonged since only one of the two fascicules of the left bundle branch is blocked.
  • This conduction disturbance does not tend to progress to more advanced degrees of bundle branch block and does not warrant any treatment per se; however, many cats with LAFB patterns are found to have cardiomyopathy. This ECG finding in conjunction with the presence of a systolic murmur warrants further diagnostics, such as thoracic radiography or echocardiography prior to general anesthesia for a dental procedure.

Answer 19

1 ECG 19 shows rapid VT.
2 • The heart rate is 300 bpm. There are no P waves associated with the ventricular beats and there is one fusion beat (circled) present, which helps differentiate this rhythm from a supraventricular arrhythmia. The ventricular complexes are wide and bizarre and "upright" in appearance (positive QRS deflection in leads II, III, and aVF). The arrow indicates a normal sinus beat ("capture beat"), which briefly captured control of the heart rhythm.
  • The most likely underlying cause of the ECG findings is arrhythmogenic right ventricular cardiomyopathy (ARVC). The presence of the "upright" VPC morphology in lead II is common in Boxer dogs with ARVC. Rapid VT can cause reduced cardiac output and blood pressure, and clinical signs such as weakness or syncope are common.
  • For acute life-threating VT, intravenous lidocaine (2 mg/kg bolus, up to a cumulative dose of 6–8 mg/kg) can be administered in an attempt to convert to sinus rhythm. The first choice for oral antiarrhythmic therapy for treatment of symptomatic VT in most dogs, including Boxers with ARVC, is sotalol.
  • Ambulatory ECG monitoring (Holter) is useful to determine the effect of therapy on frequency and severity of ventricular arrhythmias or to detect VPCs in dogs with only intermittent arrhythmias.

19

Question 20

ECG 20a was recorded in a 9-year-old female spayed Siberian Husky. ECG 20b was recorded from a geriatric Cocker Spaniel.

1 What are the findings in **ECG 20a** (50 mm/s; 5 mm/mV) and **ECG 20b** (25 mm/s; 10 mm/mV)?
2 What is the clinical significance of these ECGs?

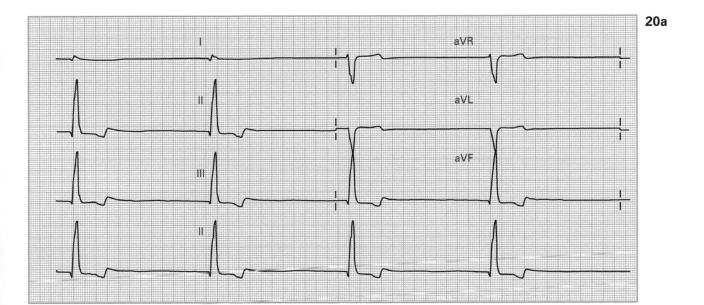

20a

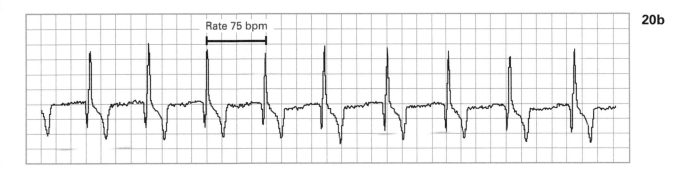

20b

Answer 20

1 ECGs **20a** and **20b** show atrial standstill.

2 • The heart rate in **ECG 20a** is 48 bpm and heart rate in **ECG 20b** is 75 bpm. In both ECGs, the rhythm is regular.

- There is an absence of P waves. The QRS complexes in **ECG 20a** are wide, indicating they are likely ventricular in origin. The slow rate and absence of normal sinus beats are consistent with a ventricular escape rhythm. The QRS complexes in **ECG 20b** are narrow indicating they are likely supraventricular in origin.

- The lack of P waves is most consistent with atrial standstill. Atrial standstill can be secondary to a degenerative atrial myopathy or secondary to severe electrolyte abnormalities, such as hyperkalemia.

- The degenerative atrial myopathy is typified by loss of functional atrial myocytes and atrial fibrosis, and atrial standstill is usually permanent. This condition was suspected in the case of **ECG 20a**.

- Hyperkalemia can be secondary to metabolic disease (i.e., diabetic ketoacidosis), endocrine disease (i.e., hypoadrenocorticism), renal failure, or reperfusion injury that sometimes accompanies feline aortic thromboembolism. In the case of **ECG 20b**, the dog had hypoadrenocorticism and a serum K^+ of 10 mmol/l (10 mEq/l). Correction of hyperkalemia (e.g., diuresis, glucose, insulin, and so on) can restore normal sinus rhythm.

Question 21

ECG recorded in a 1-year-old dog under anesthesia for a routine ovariohysterectomy.

1 What are the findings in **ECG 21** (50 mm/s; 10 mm/mV)?
2 What is the clinical significance of this ECG?

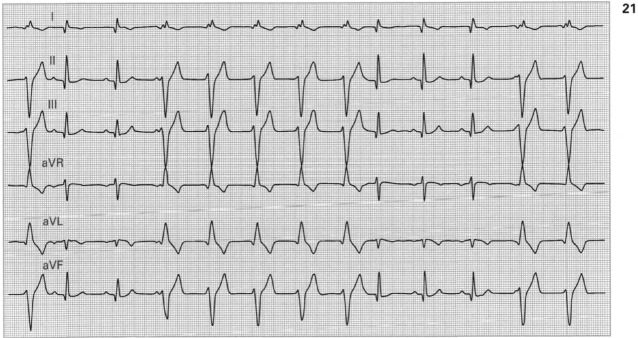

Answer 21

1 ECG 21 shows accelerated idioventricular rhythm.
   - This rhythm occurs when the discharge rates of the sinus node and another ectopic pacemaker site (nodal or ventricular) approximate each other. In this example, when the sinus rate is slightly slower than the ventricular rate, the ventricular rate "takes over." The R–R interval of the sinus complexes (blue arrow) is 460 ms (heart rate of 130 bpm) and the interval of the ventricular complexes (black arrow) is shorter at 420 ms (143 bpm). Therefore, the ventricular rate is "accelerated" and becomes the dominant rhythm until the sinus rate increases and recaptures control of the heart rate later in the strip. This arrhythmia is commonly seen in patients under anesthesia or animals with significant systemic disease.
   - Generally, no therapy is required as the sinus and ectopic pacemaker rate approximate each other. Usually, slow ventricular rhythms do not result in hemodynamic consequences and are not a significant risk for degeneration into ventricular fibrillation; however, if the ventricular rate is very fast (typically >180 bpm), antiarrhythmic treatment may be necessary.

21

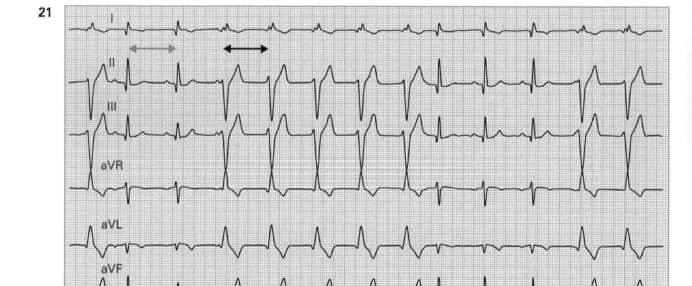

Question 22
ECG recorded in an 11-year-old Irish Setter.

1 What are the findings in **ECG 22a** (25 mm/s; 5 mm/mV)?
2 What is the clinical significance of this ECG?

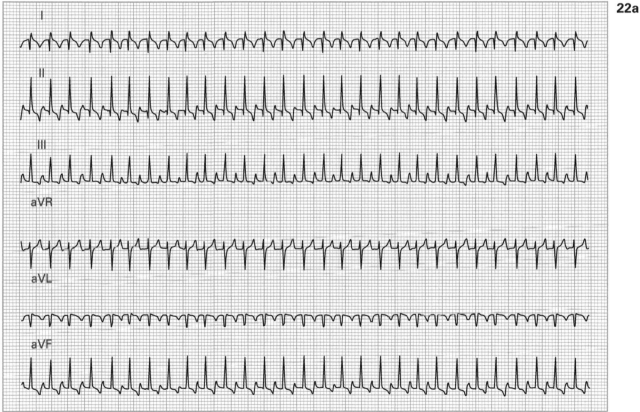

22a

Answer 22

1 **ECG 22a** shows SVT.

2 • The heart rate is 250 bpm. The rhythm is regular. The heart rate is fast enough such that the P waves in front of each QRS complex occur immediately at the end of the preceding beat's T wave. The amplitude and duration of the P and QRS complexes are normal. The MEA is normal.

  • SVT describes a rapid and usually regular rhythm that originates from either the atria or AV nodal junction. These rhythms can be due to rapid firing of ectopic foci or re-entrant rhythms. SVT can be differentiated from sinus tachycardia by: (1) its persistence despite the patient being calm or unstressed; and (2) sudden cessation secondary to vagal maneuvers or pharmacologic intervention. Many cases of SVT will have underlying cardiac disease.

  • Depending on the origin of the rhythm (atria or AV junction), the P wave configuration can be normal or altered. The QRS configuration is usually normal except in cases of aberrant conduction such as concurrent bundle branch block.

  • There is typically one P wave for every QRS complex; however, in cases of SVT and AV nodal block, the ratio of P waves to QRS complexes may be <1 (**ECG 22b**).

  • The key points are identification of a rapid rhythm with normal QRS configuration.

22b

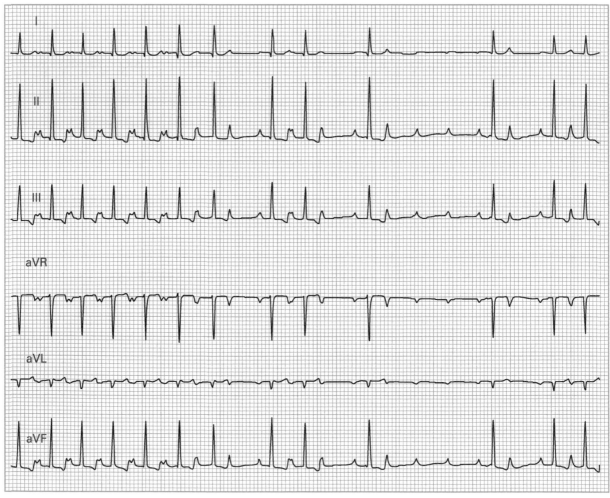

Question 23

ECG recorded in 11-year-old male castrated cat that was scheduled to have a dental cleaning. An arrhythmia and a 3/6 systolic sternal murmur was ausculted.

1 What are the findings in **ECG 23** (50 mm/s; 10 mm/mV)?
2 What is the clinical significance of this ECG?

23

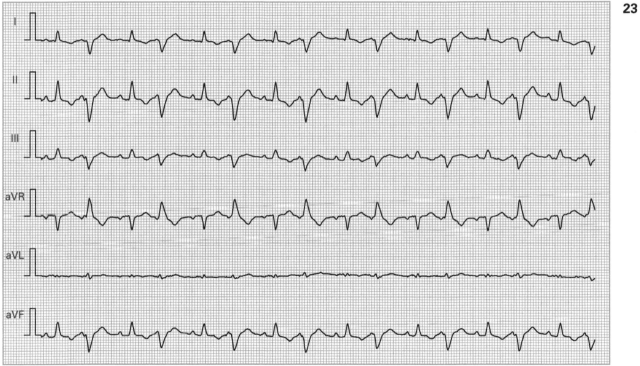

Answer 23

1 **ECG 23** shows ventricular bigeminy (sinus beat followed by a ventricular beat).

2 • The QRS complex of the ventricular beat (circled) is wide and bizarre and has a negative deflection. There are no P waves associated with these beats. Notice that the sinus beats all have P waves preceding the QRS complex (arrows).

  • The most common cause for ventricular arrhythmias in cats is cardiomyopathy and further diagnostics, such as echocardiography, are recommended. This patient was diagnosed with hypertrophic obstructive cardiomyopathy.

  • Other common diseases that can cause or exacerbate myocardial hypertrophy and associated ventricular arrhythmias include systemic hypertension and hyperthyroidism. Blood pressure and thyroid levels should both be acquired in cats with ventricular arrhythmias.

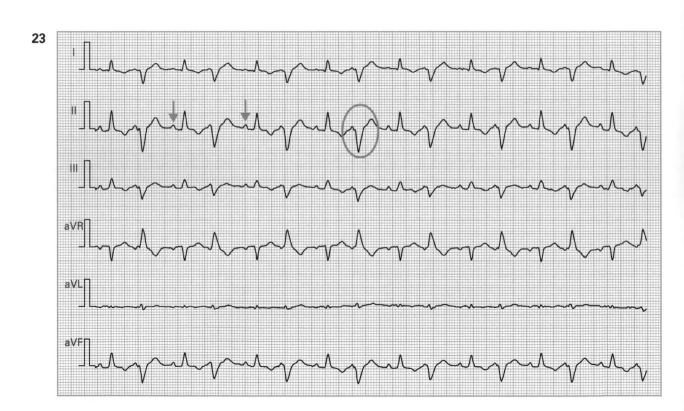

Question 24

ECG recorded from a 12-year-old Poodle dog that presented for respiratory distress.

1 What are the findings in **ECG 24** (50 mm/s, 10 mm/mV)?
2 What is the clinical significance of this ECG?

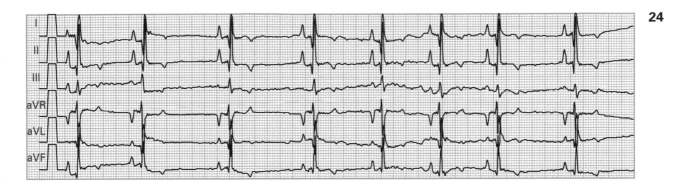

24

Question 25

ECG recording from a 15-year-old Pug dog under anesthesia.

1 What are the findings in **ECG 25** (25 mm/s; 10 mm/mV)?
2 What is the clinical significance of this ECG?

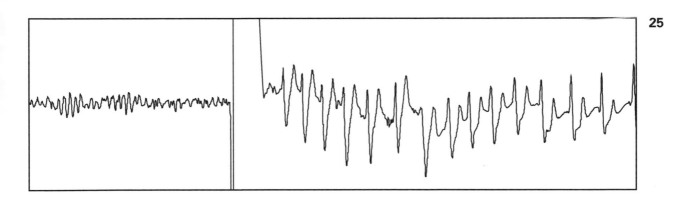

25

Answer 24

1 ECG 24 shows sinus arrhythmia and criteria for atrial enlargement.
2 • The heart rate is ~100 bpm. The P waves are tall and peaked in leads I, II, and aVF. The amplitude of the P wave in lead II is 0.5 mV (normal: <0.4 mV). A tall P wave is often referred to as "P pulmonale" despite the fact that tall P waves can be detected in both cases of left or right atrial enlargement.
   • At times, tall P waves are seen in patients with pulmonary disease, right ventricular hypertrophy, and pulmonary hypertension (cor pulmonale).

Answer 25

1 ECG 25 shows ventricular fibrillation (VF) followed by electrical defibrillation, a wide complex tachycardia, and finally a more narrow complex tachycardia.
   • Section A shows VF, recognized by the low voltage undulating baseline and absence of distinct P waves or QRS complexes. During VF, cardiac output and arterial blood pressure are absent and immediate intervention is indicated. The arrow shows delivery of a transthoracic defibrillation shock of 50 Joules with a biphasic defibrillator. The ECG trace disappears during the shock application due to the high current flow.
   • Approximately 1 second following the shock, a wide complex tachycardia at 230 bpm appears and is likely VT. Despite the abnormal nature of this initial postshock rhythm, it immediately provided a coordinated cardiac contraction and blood pressure, which is vital. The wide complex tachycardia begins to assume a narrow complex morphology toward the end of the strip and likely represents resumption of a supraventricular rhythm.

25

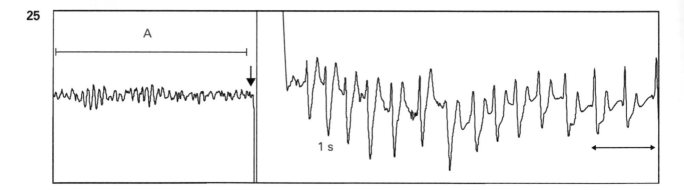

External electrical defibrillation is the treatment of choice in cases of VF. In dogs, a dose of 2–3 J/kg for external biphasic defibrillation is recommended. Direct current shocks are delivered to the heart in order to depolarize uniformly and simultaneously a critical mass of the excitable myocardium. The objectives are to interfere with all arrhythmia mechanisms and to allow the normal cardiac pacemakers to assume the role of primary pacemaker. Failure to defibrillate or immediate recurrence of VF are an indication to repeat defibrillation with a higher shock energy setting or more a optimized defibrillation set-up. Successful defibrillation depends on two key factors: (1) duration between onset of fibrillation and defibrillation, and (2) the metabolic condition of the myocardium. The goal is to use the minimum amount of energy required to overcome the threshold of defibrillation. Excessive energy can cause myocardial injury and worse arrhythmias. A large paddle-to-chest ratio, optimal paddle position on the thorax over the myocardium, firm contact pressure, and shaved chest and adequate conduction (using either disposable pads or electrode gel) all contribute to lower impedance, which allows the use of lower energy shocks.

During VF, blood flow to and from the heart ceases, resulting in rapid oxygen depletion of the myocardium. Thus, cardiopulmonary resuscitation involving chest compressions and ventilation are important while preparing the electric defibrillator or between failed defibrillation attempts. Antiarrhythmics as a means to defibrillate are rarely effective, as perfusion of the myocardium is absent during VF.

Question 26

ECG recorded from a 2-year-old Labrador Retriever that presents to the emergency service for a syncopal episode. An arrhythmia was ausculted on presentation.

1 What are the findings in **ECG 26** (50 mm/s; 10 mm/mV)?
2 What is the clinical significance of this ECG?

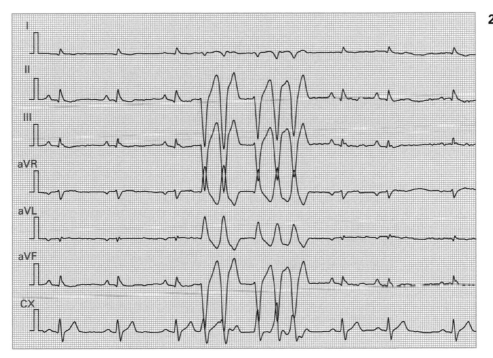

26

Answer 26

1 ECG 26 shows paroxysmal rapid VT.
2 • The maximum instantaneous heart rate of the VT is 380 bpm.
  • "R-on-T" phenomenon is present. The "R-on-T" phenomenon" is the superimposition of an ectopic beat QRS complex on the T wave of a preceding beat (arrows) due to the rapid rate of the VT. There is short pause between the first ventricular couplet and the next ventricular triplet. It is believed that these short–long intervals during VT can predispose to the onset of VF, which is a terminal rhythm unless successfully defibrillated.
  • In addition, the sinus beat QRS complexes are of low amplitude.

26

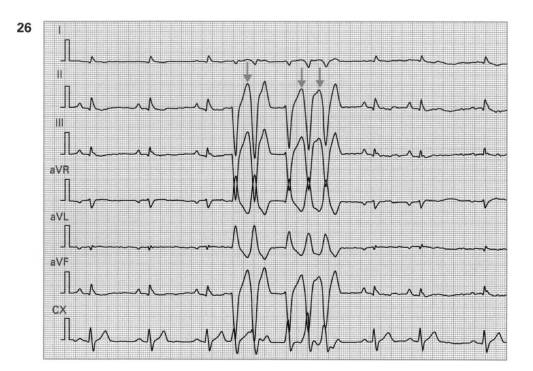

Rapid VT is uncommon in young dogs. Certain dog breeds are predisposed to a juvenile onset of cardiomyopathy and arrhythmias (such as Boxer, Doberman, Portuguese Water, and German Shepherd dogs). In this case, myocarditis was suspected due to elevated serum cardiac troponin (cTnI) concentration (13.5 ng/ml, normal: 0–0.11 ng/ml). cTnI is a highly sensitive and specific biomarker of myocardial injury and necrosis. In humans with myocardial infarction, sepsis, or traumatic myocardial injury, cTnI is used to aid in a diagnosis of cardiac injury and to provide prognostic information. cTnI is elevated in dogs and cats with a variety of diseases including myocarditis, cardiomyopathy, pericardial disease, arrhythmias, congestive heart failure, gastric dilatation and volvulus, chemotherapy, and heatstroke, and after intensive exercise.

In this case, the absence of any of these other conditions suggested a diagnosis of myocarditis. Vector-borne diseases have been implicated in myocarditis; thus, testing for heartworm, anaplasmosis, Lyme disease, *Ehrlichia* toxoplasmosis, *Neospira* spp., *Bartonella* spp., and leptospirosis can be considered. The underlying cause is often not identified. The cTnI half-life is ~2 hours in the dog, thus serial measurements might be helpful in determining the presence of either ongoing or resolving myocardial injury.

Treatment of suspected myocarditis depends on whether an underlying cause has been identified. Anti-inflammatory therapy is controversial. Many patients receive empiric doxycycline and/or clindamycin treatment. If the VT causes clinical signs such as syncope, sotalol (2–3 mg/kg PO q12h) is prescribed. Ideally, a pre- and post-treatment Holter examination is acquired to assess the efficacy of the antiarrhythmic therapy.

Question 27

ECG recorded from a 7-year-old Shar-Pei that presents for exercise intolerance.

1 What are the findings in **ECG 27** (50 mm/s; 10 mm/mV)?
2 What is the clinical significance of this ECG?

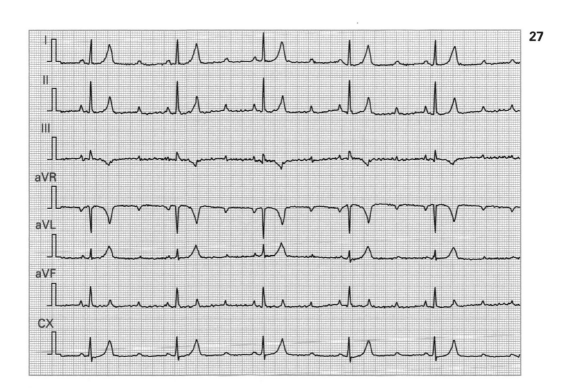

27

Answer 27

1 **ECG 27** shows second-degree AV nodal block.

2 • The ventricular rate is approximately 75 bpm. There are P waves present without a subsequent QRS complex. There are three P waves (arrows) for every QRS complex, and the AV block can be further described using a ratio of P waves to QRS complexes, or 3:1. One of the P waves is buried in the T wave. In AV block with 2:1 conduction ratio or higher, prolongation of the PR interval before the block is impossible to observe so Mobitz type I or II labeling cannot be performed, and this form of second-degree AV block is often referred to as "high grade."

• The exercise intolerance in this case might be explained by the AV block and resulting bradycardia. As explained in **ECG 9** (p. 54), an atropine response test can be performed to help differentiate increased vagal tone versus intrinsic AV nodal disease as a cause of the AV block. In most instances of high-grade second-degree AV block, AV node disease is present. Patients experiencing even a partial response to atropine may be candidates for medical management with vagolytic drugs (e.g., probantheline bromide) and/or a sympathomimetic drug (e.g., albuterol, theophylline).

• Second-degree AV block can progress to third-degree AV block, and further diagnostics include Holter recording to screen for other periods of AV block. Artificial pacemaker implantation can be used to treat symptomatic high-grade or third-degree AV block.

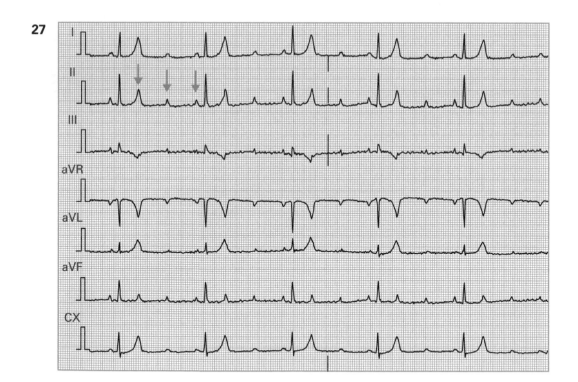

27

Question 28

ECG recorded from a 10-year-old Labrador Retriever presented to the veterinary hospital for a routine dental prophylaxis.

1 What are the findings in **ECG 28** (50 mm/s; 10 mm/mV)?
2 What is the clinical significance of this ECG?

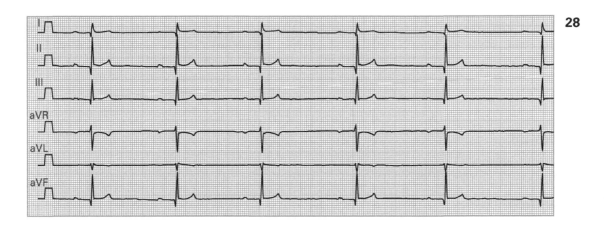

28

Question 29

ECG recorded in a 10-year-old mixed breed dog.

1 What are the findings in **ECG 29** (25 mm/s; 10 mm/mV)?
2 What is the clinical significance of this ECG?

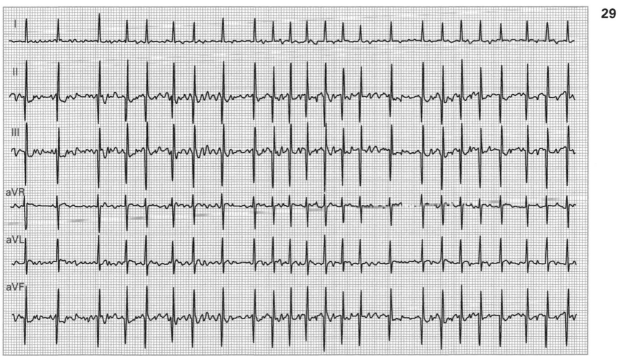

29

Answer 28

1 **ECG 28** shows a normal sinus rhythm and first-degree AV nodal block.
2 • The heart rate is 70 bpm. The P waves and QRS complexes are normal in morphology. The PR interval is 160 ms (normal: 60–130 ms) and consistent with a diagnosis of first-degree AV block.
  • First-degree AV block has no clinical sequelae unless it progresses to a more advanced form (i.e., second- or third-degree AV block). The exact etiology of AV block is often undetermined but can be due to high resting vagal tone, degeneration or infiltration of the AV node, or infectious or inflammatory disease. A first-degree AV block can also be an incidental finding in a healthy dog. Drugs that reduce or slow AV nodal conduction such as beta-blockers, digoxin, or calcium-channel blockers can exacerbate this conduction delay and result in more advanced forms of AV block. Opioids increase vagal tone and it might be best to avoid these drugs during the anesthesia protocol.

Answer 29

1 **ECG 29** shows atrial fibrillation (AF).
2 • The average heart rate is ~210 bpm. The rhythm is irregularly irregular and there are no P waves. The QRS complexes are narrow and of supraventricular morphology. The baseline displays small atrial fibrillatory waves (f waves).
  • AF usually occurs in the presence of advanced cardiac disease, such as mitral valve disease or dilated cardiomyopathy. In these instances, the ventricular rate is typically rapid, thus requiring medications (e.g., digoxin, diltiazem, and/or atenolol) to slow conduction through the AV node and slow the rate. Spontaneous conversion back to sinus rhythm is rare. In some large breed dogs, AF can occur without any identifiable underlying cardiac disease (lone AF). In this instance, the ventricular rate is usually slow and might not require medication. Conversion of lone AF back to sinus rhythm using electric cardioversion (see **ECG 5**, p. 50) or antiarrhythmic medications (amiodarone) is possible.
  • The key points are the irregularity of the ventricular rhythm, lack of P waves, the normal morphology of the QRS complexes indicating a supraventricular origin, and the rapid ventricular rate.

Question 30

ECG recorded from a 6-year-old male castrated Boston Terrier presented with a 4/6 left-sided systolic apical murmur.

1 What are the findings in **ECG 30** (50 mm/s; 10 mm/mV)?
2 What is the clinical significance of this ECG?

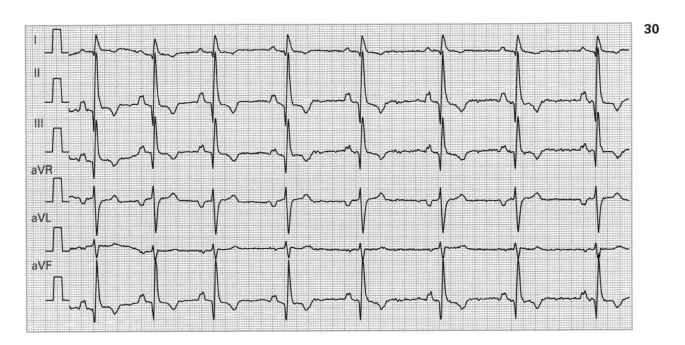

30

Question 31

ECG recorded from a 10-year-old West Highland White Terrier with progressive weakness and syncope.

1 What are the findings in **ECG 31** (50 mm/s; 10 mm/mV)?
2 What is the clinical significance of this ECG?

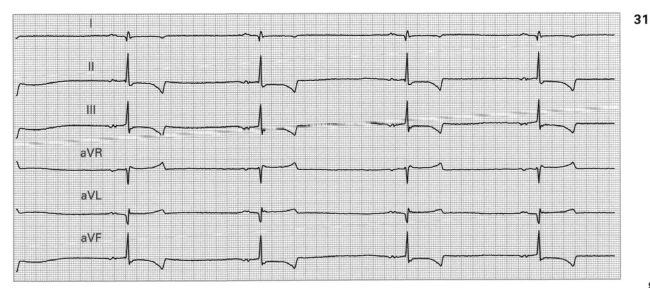

31

Answer 30

1 ECG 30 shows sinus arrhythmia and criteria for atrial enlargement.
2 • The heart rate is 90 bpm. There are wide and notched (bifid) P waves in leads II, III, and aVF. The P wave duration in lead II is 60 ms (normal: <40 ms). A wide and notched P wave is also referred to as "P mitrale" despite the fact that tall P waves can be detected in cases of both left or right atrial enlargement.
  • Atrial enlargement is associated with volume overload and increased atrial size, as for example occurs with degenerative mitral or tricuspid valve disease or cardiomyopathy. ECG detection of atrial enlargement is relatively insensitive but usually specific in both cats and dogs. This patient had severe left atrial enlargement due to advanced degenerative mitral valve disease.

Answer 31

1 ECG 31 shows sinus bradycardia and QT interval prolongation.
2 • The heart rate is ~45 bpm. The PR interval is mildly prolonged at 140 ms, indicating first-degree AV block. The P wave is notched and low voltage in lead II. The QRS duration is normal, but the QT interval is markedly prolonged at 360 ms (normal: 150–250 ms, depending on heart rate). The QT interval is measured from the beginning of the QRS complex to the end of the T wave and represents the total duration of electrical depolarization and subsequent repolarization of the ventricular myocardium. The QT interval is inversely related to the heart rate.
  • Long QT syndromes are caused by abnormal ionic current flow during repolarization. Various drugs are a common cause of a long QT interval, including the class IA antiarrhythmic agents, including quinidine, procainamide, and disopyramide, and class III antiarrhythmic agents, including sotalol and amiodarone. A number of noncardiac drugs have also been reported to prolong QT interval, including cisapride, phenothiazines, haloperidol, tricyclic antidepressants, antimicrobial agents (erythromycin, chloroquine, and trimethoprim–sulfamethoxazole), and antifungal agents (ketoconazole and itraconazole).
  • Long QT intervals predispose to the development of polymorphic ventricular arrhythmias, (torsade de pointes; see **ECG 4**, p. 48).

Question 32

ECG recorded in a 13-year-old female domestic shorthair cat.

1 What are the findings in **ECG 32** (50 mm/s; 10 mm/mV)?
2 What is the clinical significance of this ECG?

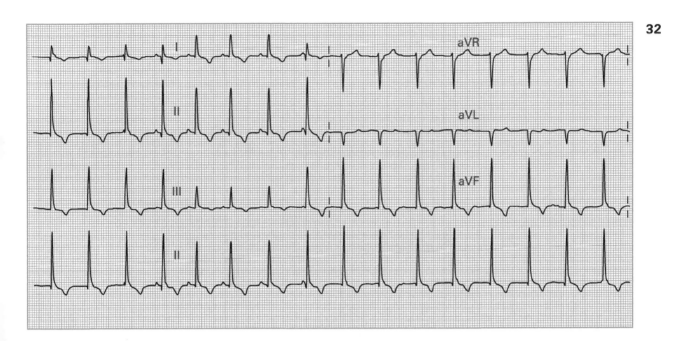

32

Answer 32

1 ECG 32 shows an accelerated junctional rhythm and evidence of left heart enlargement.

2 • The average heart rate is 185 bpm. The rhythm is slightly irregular.

- Two different QRS complex morphologies are noted. P waves can be intermittently seen in front of QRS complexes of normal duration (arrows), and these beats appear to be sinus beats (heart rate 195–214 bpm). Other QRS complexes also with narrow duration but greater amplitude (arrowheads) do not have a P wave associated with them, and these beats are most likely an accelerated junctional rhythm (heart rate 195 bpm).

- The junctional (as opposed to ventricular) origin of the accelerated beats is suggested by the narrow QRS complex.

- The amplitude of the sinus beat QRS complexes is increased at 1.9 mV (normal <0.9 mV) indicating left ventricular enlargement.

- Accelerated junctional rhythms compete with the sinus node for control of the heart rate. When the sinus rate speeds up above the rate of the junctional rhythm, the sinus rate captures control of the rhythm. When the sinus rate slows below that of the accelerated junctional rate, the junctional rhythm captures control of the rhythm.

- Accelerated junctional rhythms can occur secondary to underlying cardiomyopathy, as well as secondary to extracardiac disease such as trauma, hypoxia, electrolyte abnormalities, and drugs.

32

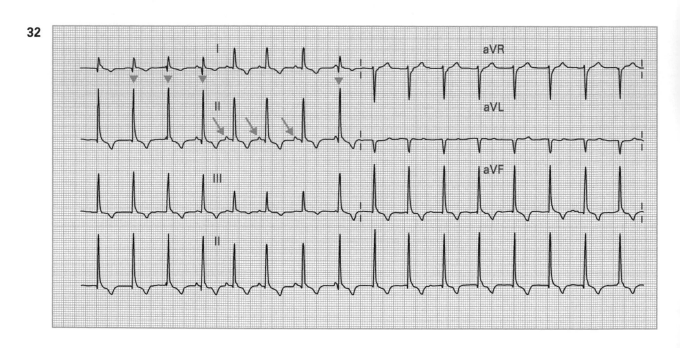

Question 33

ECG recorded from a 3-year-old Welsh Springer Spaniel that presents for exercise intolerance.

1 What are the findings in **ECG 33** (50 mm/s; 10 mm/mV)?
2 What is the clinical significance of this ECG?

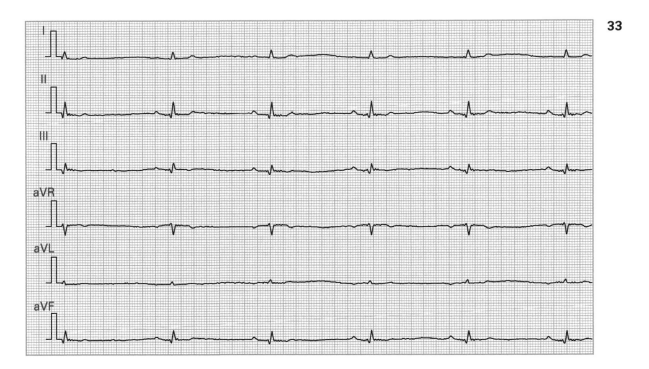

33

Question 34

ECG recorded from a 5-year-old cat with a heart murmur.

1 What are the findings in **ECG 34** (50 mm/s; 10 mm/mV)?
2 What is the clinical significance of this ECG?

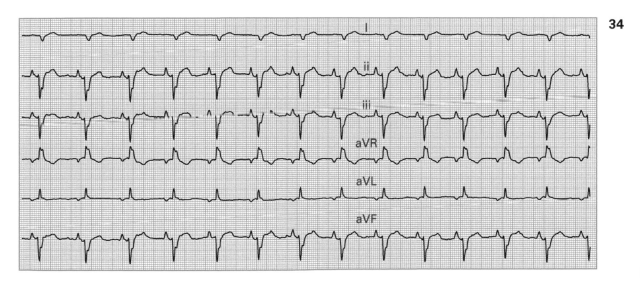

34

Answer 33

1 ECG 33 shows sinus arrhythmia, first-degree AV nodal block, and low amplitude QRS complexes.
2 • The heart rate is ~80 bpm. There is a prolonged PR interval of 140 ms, which is indicative of first-degree AV block. The amplitude of the R waves is <1.0 mV in leads I, II, III, and aVF, which is unusual for a medium or large breed dog.
  • Conditions associated with low amplitude QRS complexes include a variety of cardiac and extracardiac causes. Pericardial effusion is the most common cardiac cause of low amplitude QRS complexes. Other causes include cardiomyopathy, cardiac neoplasia, constrictive pericarditis, and myocarditis.
  • Extracardiac causes are due to the pathology of organs and tissues surrounding the heart. Causes include peritoneopericardial diaphragmatic hernia, pneumomediastinum, pneumothorax, pneumonia, and obesity. This patient had a peritoneopericardial diaphragmatic hernia that was surgically corrected as it was causing clinical signs of exercise intolerance. The first-degree AV block is an incidental finding and of no clinical consequence.

Answer 34

1 ECG 34 shows sinus rhythm and right bundle branch block (RBBB).
2 • The heart rate is 150 bpm. The duration of the QRS is prolonged at 80 ms (normal: <40 ms). The QRS complexes in leads I, II, III, and aVF are negative and the MEA is shifted to the right at −120°. This shift in MEA occurs because conduction is blocked down the right bundle, so that the depolarization travels rapidly down the left bundle branch activating the left ventricle first, followed by right ventricular depolarization. The right ventricular depolarization is prolonged due to slower conduction from myocyte to myocyte instead of the rapidly conducting Purkinje system. This results in the late and dominant S wave in the aforementioned leads. There is a notch in the QRS complex, which is commonly seen in cases of RBBB.
  • RBBB occurs either as a consequence of conduction system disease in the right bundle branch or can be an incidental finding in a healthy animal, particularly in dogs. Rarely, RBBB is associated with severe right ventricular hypertrophy secondary to a pressure overload condition such as pulmonic stenosis. More commonly, such conditions produce a right axis shift but without excessive prolongation of conduction time.
  • Due to the delayed activation of the right ventricle, RBBB may cause a prolonged right ventricular ejection time, thus resulting in delayed closure of the pulmonic valve, which may be ausculted as a split second heart sound.

Question 35

ECG recorded from an 8-year-old Doberman Pinscher with dilated cardiomyopathy.

1 What are the findings in **ECG 35** (50 mm/s; 10 mm/mV)?
2 What is the clinical significance of this ECG?

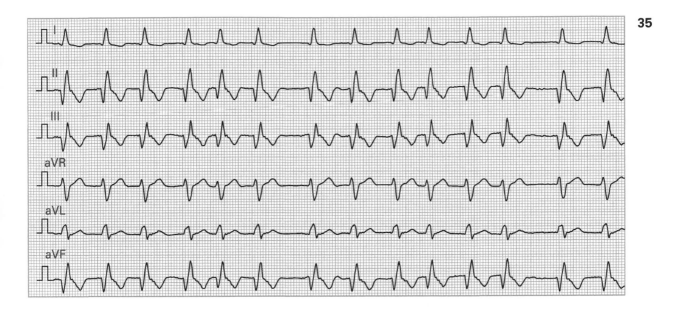

35

Question 36

ECG recorded from an 8-year-old Doberman Pinscher with a history of syncope.

1 What are the findings in **ECG 36** (50 mm/s; 10 mm/mV)?
2 What is the clinical significance of this ECG?

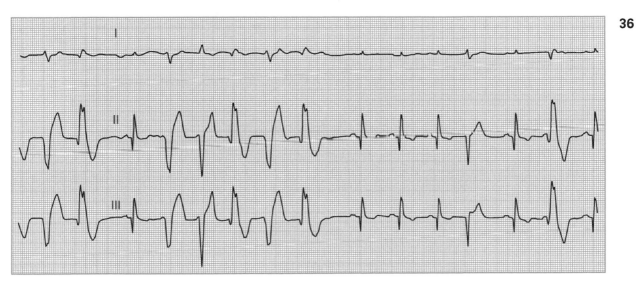

36

Answer 35

1 ECG 35 shows AF and a LBBB morphology.
2 • The heart rate is ~185 bpm. The rhythm is irregularly irregular. The QRS duration is prolonged (>80 ms) due to a wide Q and R wave.
  • The diagnosis of an LBBB is made based on a normal MEA of the QRS complex with increased duration of the QRS.
  • AF is a common sequela to atrial dilation associated with advanced dilated cardiomyopathy. Due to the absence of P waves and the LBBB morphology, one may be inclined to make a diagnosis of VT in this ECG. The key feature to recognize AF with a LBBB is the irregularity of the rhythm; VT is usually more regular.
  • AF in the setting of advanced myocardial failure is typically associated with tachycardia and can lead to exacerbation of heart failure signs, such as ascites or pulmonary edema.

Answer 36

1 ECG 36 shows polymorphic VT.
2 • Five sinus beats (black arrows) are seen. The other complexes are wide and bizarre compared to the normal sinus beats, indicating a ventricular origin. A short period of VT consisting of five ventricular premature beats (blue arrows) is detected in the middle of the recording, with a heart rate of 200 bpm. The VPCs have two different and distinct morphologies (i.e., polymorphic), suggesting that they arise from two different areas within the ventricles.
  • There is one potential fusion beat (green arrow), indicating simultaneous ventricular depolarization from a sinus impulse and a ventricular ectopic impulse. The resultant QRS complex morphology is a combination of a normal sinus QRS and abnormal VPC QRS.
  • In this case, dilated cardiomyopathy was diagnosed via echocardiography and the antiarrhythmic agent sotalol was prescribed, based on the presumption that syncope was being caused by longer runs of polymorphic VT.

36

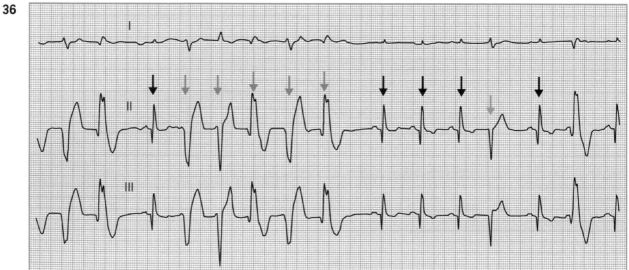

Question 37

ECG 37 was recorded in an 18-year-old cat with a history of chronic dyspnea.

1 What are the findings in **ECG 37** (50 mm/s; 10 mm/mV)?
2 What is the clinical significance of this ECG?

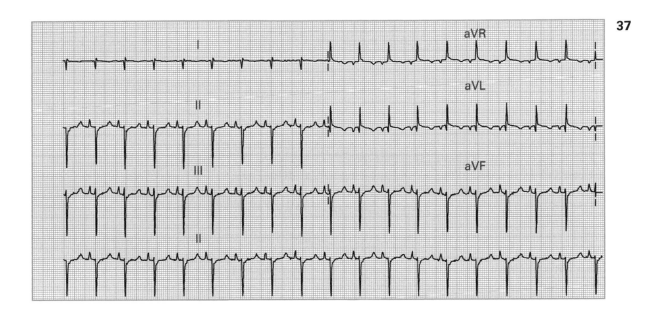

37

Question 38

ECG recorded in a 2-year-old Rottweiler, with a grade 4/6 systolic murmur.

1 What are the findings in **ECG 38** (50 mm/s; 5 mm/mV)?
2 What is the clinical significance of this ECG?

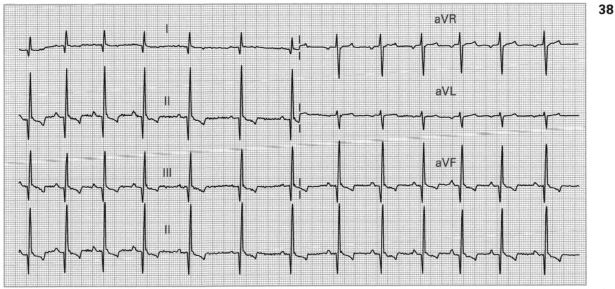

38

Answer 37

1 **ECG 37** shows a sinus rhythm and criteria for right ventricular hypertrophy.

2 • The heart rate is 215 bpm. The QRS duration is within normal limits and each is preceded by a normal P wave. There is a shift in the MEA to the right at –100°, indicated by a predominantly negative QRS morphology in leads I, II, III, and aVF.

• Right axis deviations are associated with either right ventricular hypertrophy or RBBB, with the discriminating feature being the duration of the QRS complex. QRS durations >60 ms in the cat are characteristic of RBBB (see **ECG 34**, p. 87), and durations <60 ms typical of right heart hypertrophy.

• In this cat an echocardiogram revealed marked right ventricular hypertrophy due to pulmonary hypertension and tricuspid insufficiency.

Answer 38

1 **ECG 38** shows sinus arrhythmia with criteria for left ventricular hypertrophy.

2 • The heart rate is ~150 bpm. Note that the ECG was recorded at 5 mm/mV, which results in the amplitude of the QRS complex as appearing half its actual height. The P wave amplitude is normal at 0.4 mV. The MEA is +80°, which is in the normal range. The R wave amplitude in lead II is 4.4 mV, in lead aVF is 4.6 mV, and in lead I is 1.5 mV, all of which are indicative of left ventricular hypertrophy.

• Left ventricular hypertrophy increases the magnitude of the electrical wavefront travelling through the left ventricle, resulting in an increased R wave in leads parallel with this wavefront, primarily leads II and aVF. Diseases that cause left heart hypertrophy include cardiomyopathy, valve disease, and a variety of congenital heart defects. The left heart hypertrophy pattern is not specific to any one disease or cause, and further diagnostics such as thoracic radiography or echocardiography are warranted.

• In this case, echocardiography revealed congenital subaortic stenosis and resulting concentric left ventricular hypertrophy.

Question 39

ECG recorded from a 1-year-old cat presented to the emergency service with a history of syncope and having just received a calcium-channel blocker (diltiazem).

1 What are the findings in **ECG 39a** (25 mm/s, 20 mm/mV)?
2 What is the clinical significance of this ECG?

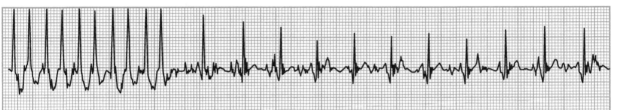

39a

Answer 39

1 **ECG 39a** shows an SVT converting into sinus rhythm.

2 • The initial section of **ECG 39a** shows a narrow complex tachycardia at a rate of 300 bpm. The QRS complexes are tall and narrow and therefore the arrhythmia is presumed to be supraventricular in origin, despite the fact that P waves cannot be readily identified. The heart rate is rapid enough that any P waves will be buried in the preceding T wave. Diltiazem, a calcium-channel blocker, was administered and the SVT terminated abruptly followed by a sinus rhythm with a heart rate of 125 bpm.

 • This ECG demonstrates the difficulty in discerning VT from SVT when the heart rate is very rapid. A differential diagnosis for the arrhythmia is VT, as the QRS complexes during the tachycardia do not look exactly like the QRS complexes during sinus rhythm. The response to diltiazem, however, strongly suggests that this was a SVT, as calcium-channel blockers are effective at terminating SVTs but are not effective at treating ventricular arrhythmias.

The cat from **ECG 39a** was stabilized and a subsequent ECG was recorded several hours later (**ECG 39b**). The ECG shows sinus rhythm with a heart rate of 200 bpm. The PR interval is unusually short (40 ms; normal: 50–90 ms), resulting in a P wave that appears very close to the QRS complex. This finding (ventricular pre-excitation) coupled with the history of SVT is suggestive of the presence of an accessory AV pathway. Accessory pathways (APs) are extra-AV nodal pathways situated between the atria and the ventricles and allow the cardiac impulse to travel directly from the atria to the ventricles while bypassing the AV node. Normal conduction via the AV node is also present. In ventricular pre-excitation, the AP reaches the ventricle prior to AV nodal impulses and "pre-excites" the ventricle, causing early activation and a short PR interval. The normal conduction via the AV node fuses with the pre-excitation impulse and can result in a QRS complex with a slurred upstroke, called a *delta wave*.

Pre-excitation by itself has little clinical consequence; however, the presence of the AP along with the AV node creates a circuit of conduction tissue that promotes development of SVT. SVT as seen in **ECG 39a** is often triggered by an atrial premature contraction. The tachycardia utilizes the AV node for forward conduction and the AP for conduction back to the atria. Drugs that block AV nodal conduction, such as diltiazem, can terminate the SVT by blocking impulse conduction through the AV node. Other antiarrhythmic drugs can selectively slow conduction in the AP and can also be effective at terminating the tachycardia. Cessation of tachycardia that is resistant to medical therapy requires interventional procedures such as catheter ablation using radiofrequency energy to destroy (ablate) the accessory pathway.

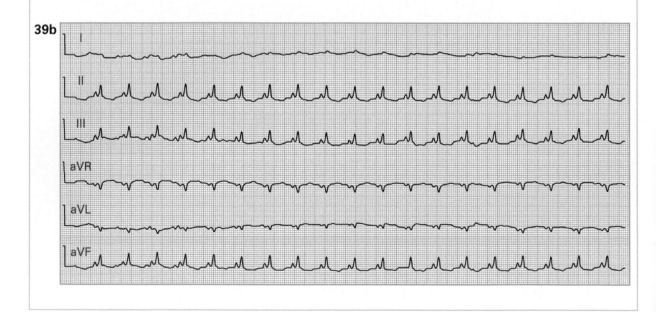

39b

Question 40

ECG recorded from a 5-month-old German Shepherd dog with a continuous murmur.

1 What are the findings in **ECG 40** (50 mm/s; 5 mm/mV)?
2 What is the clinical significance of this ECG?

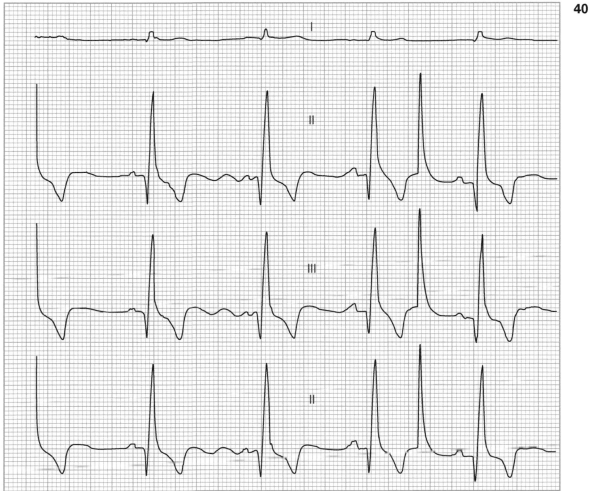

40

Answer 40

1 **ECG 40** shows sinus rhythm with criteria for left ventricular enlargement and a motion artifact.

2 • The heart rate is 115 bpm. The P waves are normal in amplitude and duration. Note that the ECG was performed with a sensitivity setting of 5 mm/mV, which results in complexes half their normal size. Thus, the R wave amplitude is increased at 4.0 mV (normal: <3.0 mV in large breed dogs) and the QRS duration is prolonged at 70 ms (normal: <60 ms). Both of these findings are consistent with left ventricular hypertrophy. Based on the dog's age and breed and presence of a continuous murmur, a patent ductus arteriosus is the most likely cause of the left heart hypertrophy.

• The fourth complex from the left is a result of movement artifact. At first inspection, the ECG complex appears to have a morphology similar to the surrounding QRS complexes and to arrive earlier than expected, thereby suggesting that it is a supraventricular or atrial premature beat. However, two characteristics indicate that it is an artifact. First, the "QRS complex" does not have a characteristic T wave following it similar to all the other beats, and second, the "QRS complex" is absent from lead I. It is impossible for the heart to depolarize (forming a QRS complex) and not to repolarize (forming a T wave), and it would be highly unlikely that a true QRS complex would not be detected in all leads. Based on the orientation of leads I, II, and III (see Section 1, **Fig. 1.1**), artifact generated by the left hind limb (in this case movement of the leg) will cause artifact in leads II and III, which both use the left hind limb as one pole of the ECG recording, but be absent in lead I, which uses the left and right forelimbs for its ECG recording.

• Electrocardiographic artifact is common in dogs and cats and careful inspection of the ECG is needed to avoid misinterpretation of these deflections.

Question 41

ECG recorded in an 11-year-old mixed breed dog.

1 What are the findings in **ECG 41** (50 mm/s; 10 mm/mV)?
2 What is the clinical significance of this ECG?

41

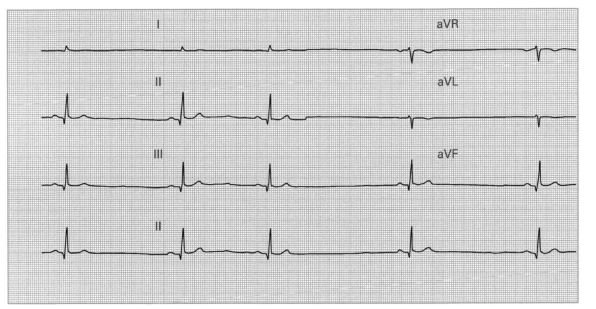

Question 42

ECG recorded from a 4-month-old German Shepherd dog under general anesthesia.

1 What are the findings in **ECG 42** (25 mm/s; 10 mm/mV)?
2 What is the clinical significance of this ECG?

42

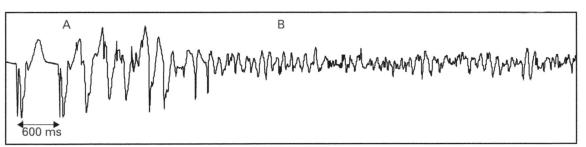

Answer 41

1 ECG 41 shows sinus bradycardia (SB).
2 • The heart rate ranges from 44 bpm to 70 bpm. The rhythm is slightly irregular.
  • There is a normal P wave, QRS complex, and T wave for every beat.
  • Causes of SB include high resting vagal tone, sinus node dysfunction, electrolyte abnormalities (i.e., hyperkalemia), central nervous system disease, hypothermia, and drugs (e.g., anesthestics, sedatives, opioids).
  • In this case, the cause of the SB is likely related to high resting vagal tone as the irregularity is suggestive of sinus arrhythmia. If so, a normal response to exercise or administration of atropine should be an increase in the heart rate and regularity. Failure to respond to these stimuli can signal underlying conduction system disease.

Answer 42

1 ECG 42 shows VT degenerating into VF.
2 • The first two QRS complexes (**A**) are the result of an artificial pacemaker with a rate of 100 bpm. The rhythm changes into a rapid and polymorphic VT, before it degenerates into VF (**B**). VF is characterized by low amplitude and disorganized electrical activity of the heart where the ECG deflections constantly change in shape, direction, and amplitude. Normal P–QRS–T waves are not discernible during VF. In this example the fibrillatory waves appear relatively coarse. Typically, the amplitude of coarse fibrillation becomes progressively lower with ever-finer oscillations detected on the ECG.
  • During VF, the ventricular muscle twitches randomly, rather than contracting in a coordinated fashion. Subsequently the ventricles fail to pump blood into the systemic and pulmonary circulation. VF causes loss of consciousness within seconds, as cardiac output totally ceases, and the rhythm is fatal if not treated immediately. External electrical defibrillation is the most successful method to terminate VF and help restore a more effective rhythm.

Question 43

ECG recorded from a 10-year-old Cocker Spaniel.

1 What are the findings in **ECG 43** (50 mm/s; 10 mm/mV)?
2 What is the clinical significance of this ECG?

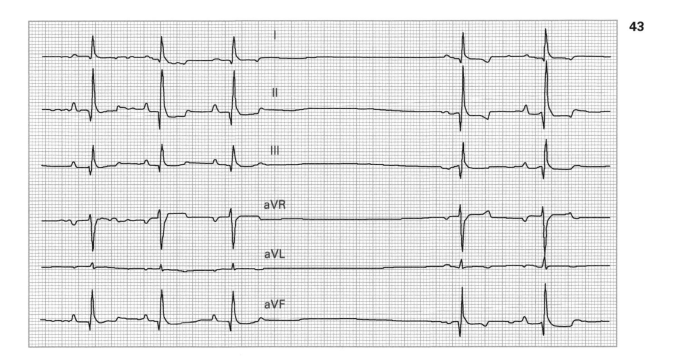

43

Question 44

ECG recorded in a 7-year-old male domestic shorthair cat.

1 What are the findings in **ECG 44** (50 mm/s; 10 mm/mV)?
2 What is the clinical significance of this ECG?

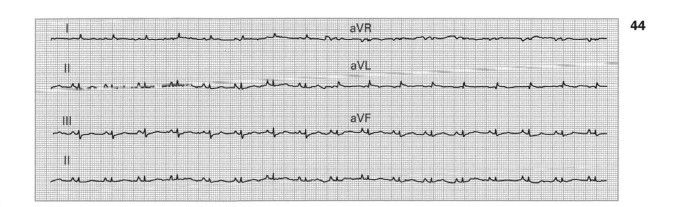

44

Answer 43

1 ECG 43 shows a junctional escape complex.
2 • The first three beats appear sinus in origin with a rate of 120 bpm. After these beats there is a period of sinus arrest/pause of approximately 1.4 seconds, followed by a junctional escape beat with a different P wave configuration. The QRS configuration of the junctional escape beat is normal.
  • Junctional escape beats occur when the rate of the sinus rhythm slows below the intrinsic rate of the junctional escape rhythm (typically 40–80 bpm). The P wave of the escape beat is typically different from that of the sinus beat, indicating its origin from the escape focus rather than the sinus node.
  • Escape rhythms should never be suppressed, rather the underlying cause of the bradycardia should be investigated.
  • The key points are normal QRS complexes with negative or altered P wave configuration occurring after periods of bradycardia or asystole.

Answer 44

1 ECG 44 shows sinus rhythm.
2 • The average heart rate is 200 bpm. The rhythm is regular with normal P (blue arrows), QRS (black arrows), and T waves (green arrows).
  • Sinus rhythm represents a normal sequence of atrial and ventricular depolarization that occurs at a normal heart rate. Beats are initiated by depolarization of the SA node, followed by atrial depolarization (P wave), AV node depolarization (PR interval), and ventricular depolarization (QRS complex) and repolarization (T wave). The normal T wave in cats is often very low voltage and may not be visualized at all.
  • In cats, the rate of sinus rhythm is typically 120–240 bpm.
  • Note that in the cat with normal sinus rhythm, the polarity of the QRS complexes is positive in leads II and aVF, indicating a normal MEA.

44

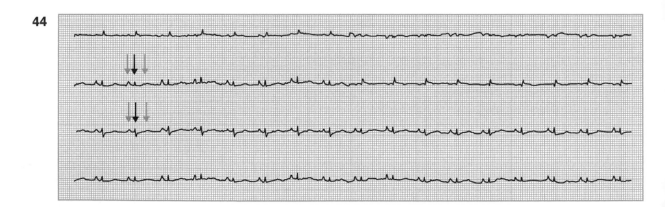

Question 45
ECG recorded in a 16-year-old male castrated domestic longhair cat with a suspected aortic thromboembolism.

1 What are the findings in **ECG 45** (50 mm/s; 10 mm/mV)?
2 What is the clinical significance of this ECG?

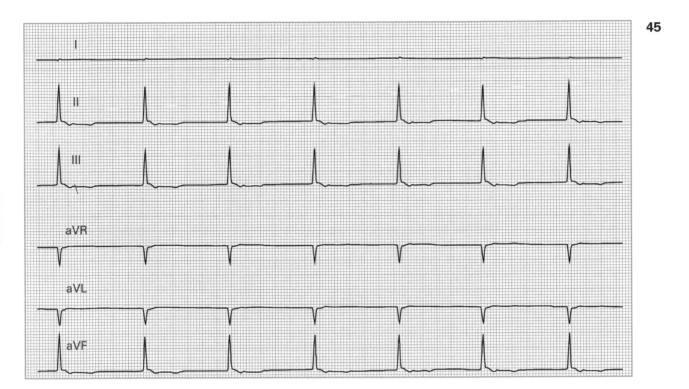

45

Question 46
ECG recorded in a 13-year-old domestic shorthair cat.

1 What are the findings in **ECG 46a** (50 mm/s; 10 mm/mV)?
2 What is the clinical significance of this ECG?

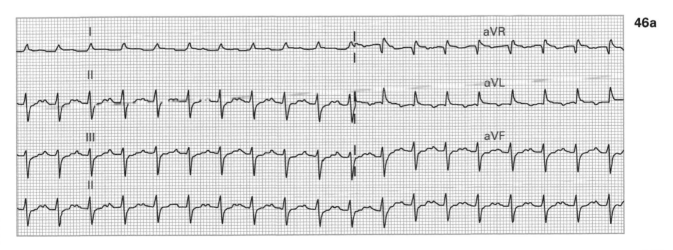

46a

Answer 45

1 ECG 45 shows atrial standstill.
2 • The heart rate is ~105 bpm and the rhythm is regular.
  • There is an absence of P waves. The QRS complexes are narrow indicating they are likely supraventricular in origin.
  • The lack of P waves, slow heart rate, and supraventricular QRS complexes are most consistent with atrial standstill. The QRS complexes are likely junctional escape beats.
  • Atrial standstill can be secondary to a degenerative atrial myopathy or secondary to severe electrolyte abnormalities, such as hyperkalemia.
  • The degenerative atrial myopathy is typified by loss of functional atrial myocytes and atrial fibrosis, and atrial standstill is usually permanent.
  • Hyperkalemia can be secondary to metabolic disease (i.e., diabetic ketoacidosis), renal failure, or reperfusion injury that sometimes accompanies feline aortic thromboembolism. Correction of hyperkalemia (e.g., diuresis, glucose, insulin, and so on) can restore normal sinus rhythm.

Answer 46

1 ECG 46a shows SVT and a left MEA shift consistent with left anterior fascicular block (LAFB).
2 • The heart rate is 300 bpm and the rhythm is regular. The QRS complexes are narrow; however, the QRS polarity is predominantly negative in leads II, III, and aVF, while positive in leads I and aVL, and is consistent with a left MEA shift (see ECG 18, p. 65).
  • There are P waves in front of each QRS complex indicating that the origin of the QRS complexes is supraventricular (rather than ventricular despite the abnormal polarity).
  • SVT can be due to underlying cardiomyopathy, hyperthyroidism, cardiac neoplasia, or drug toxicity (e.g., bronchodilators, chocolate, sympathomimetics).
  • In this case, the presence of the left axis shift is confirmed as the SVT suddenly terminates (arrows, ECG 46b) and two sinus beats (arrowheads) appear at a slower heart rate.

46b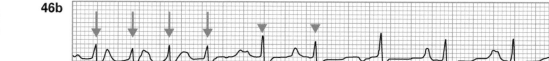

NEW GENERAL-LEVEL ECG CASES

Question 47

ECG recorded from a dog with a history of vomiting and weakness.

1 What are the findings in **ECG 47** (50 mm/sec; 10 mm/mV)?
2 What is the clinical significance of this ECG?

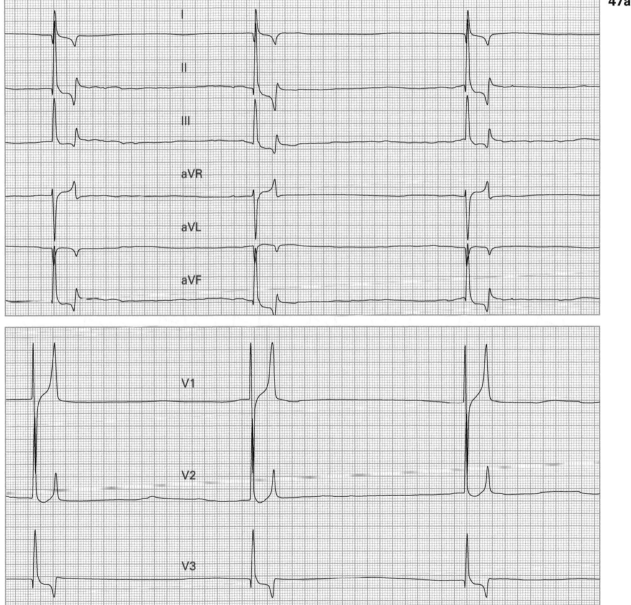

47a

Answer 47

1 **ECG 47a** shows a slow and mildly irregular ventricular heart rate at approximately 30 and 35 bpm. There are no visible P waves. The T waves in the V1 and V3 chest leads are unusually tall. The ECG rhythm is most consistent with atrial standstill. Complete (third-degree) AV nodal block is less likely due to the absence of visible P waves.

2 Atrial standstill can occur secondary to idiopathic replacement of the atrial myocardium with fibrous tissue or secondary to severe hyperkalemia, which causes failure of the atrial myocardium to depolarize and bradycardia. In this particular case, the dog's serum K^+ was markedly elevated at 8.7 mmol/L. Following treatment with IV glucose and calcium, the dog's K^+ decreased to 7.7 mmol/L, and repeat ECG revealed resumption of sinus rhythm with normal P waves and increased heart rate (**ECG 47b**). Causes of severe hyperkalemia are relatively uncommon and include ureteral obstruction, metabolic acidosis, hemolysis, complications secondary to treatment of hyperadrenocorticism, or, in this case, hypoadrenocorticism.

47b

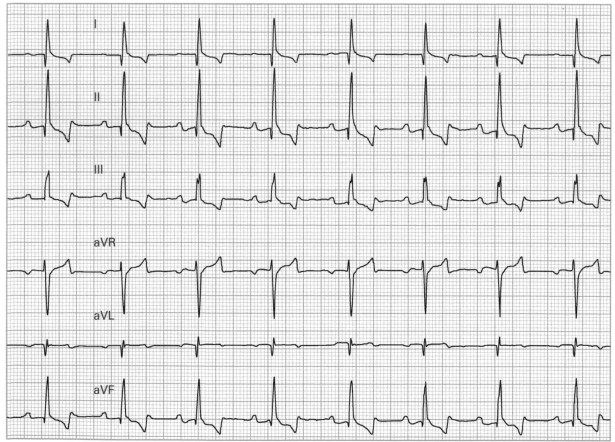

Question 48

ECG recorded from a dog with an arrhythmia detected on routine exam.

1 What are the findings in **ECG 48** (25 mm/sec; 10 mm/mV)?
2 What is the clinical significance of this ECG?

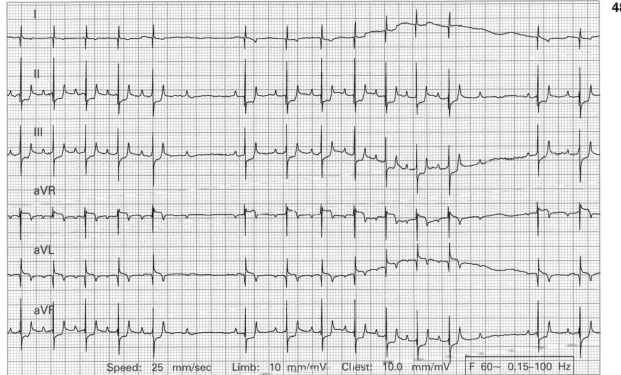

48

Answer 48

1 ECG 48 shows second-degree AV nodal block.

2 The ventricular rate during sinus rhythm is approximately 135 bpm. There are P waves without subsequent QRS complexes, indicating a failure of the sinus impulses to travel through the AV node and depolarize the ventricles.

3 The PR interval of the sinus beat preceding the dropped P waves is 0.16 seconds (4 mm × 0.04 sec/mm). This PR interval is the same as the other sinus beats and the second-degree AV nodal block is further described as type II, wherein the PR interval is not increased in the beats prior to the dropped P wave.

4 The dropped P waves are relatively infrequent and no clinical signs are necessarily expected; however, the owner should be queried further about subtle changes in the dog's activity and behavior. The presence of second-degree AV nodal block raises suspicion of underlying AV node disease. Diagnostic options include watchful waiting and recheck ECG in 3–6 months or ambulatory ECG (Holter) monitoring to better characterize the frequency and severity of the AV nodal block over a 24- or 48-hour time period.

Question 49
ECG recorded from a 7-year-old Labrador Retriever with a heart murmur.

1 What are the findings in **ECG 49a** (50 mm/sec; 10 mm/mV)?
2 What is the clinical significance of the ECG?

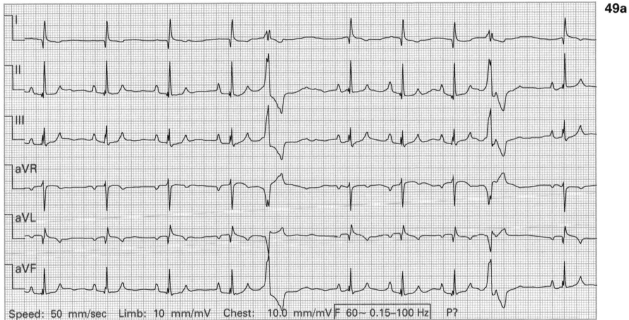

49a

Answer 49

1 ECG 49a shows sinus rhythm with a rate of 120 bpm, with two monomorphic ventricular premature beats. There is a P wave visible in the ST segment of the second ventricular premature beat (arrow) that is blocked at the AV node, likely due to retrograde depolarization of the AV node by the premature beat (arrow, ECG 49b). The QRS complexes are notched and particularly noticeable in the R wave of lead III and Q waves of leads II and aVF. The ventricular premature beats also have a notch in their R wave.

2 The presence of the ventricular premature beats could be due to underlying heart disease, such as cardiomyopathy, or due to extracardiac causes such as the presence of abdominal masses or other systemic illnesses. Notches in the QRS complex are relatively nonspecific, but have been previously associated with myocardial injury or fibrosis. The likelihood of heart disease increases with the number of leads demonstrating notching. Further diagnostics in this dog might include echocardiography, chest radiography, and investigation into the possible presence of abdominal or systemic disease. In the absence of clinical signs, specific antiarrhythmic treatment for the ventricular premature beats is likely unnecessary; however, ambulatory ECG (Holter) monitoring might be considered to further characterize the frequency and extent of any ventricular arrhythmias.

49b
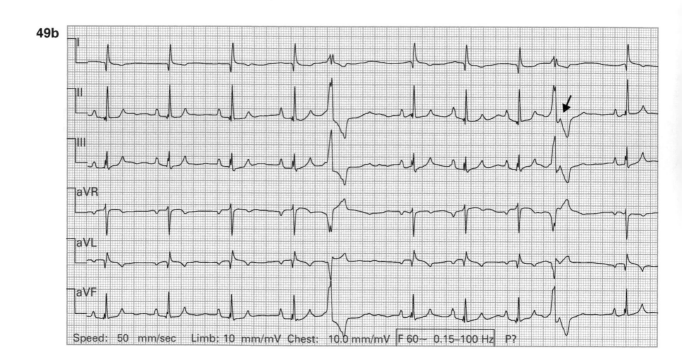

Question 50
ECG recorded from a cat.

1 What are the findings in **ECG 50a** (50 mm/sec; 10 mm/mV)?
2 What is the clinical significance of the ECG?

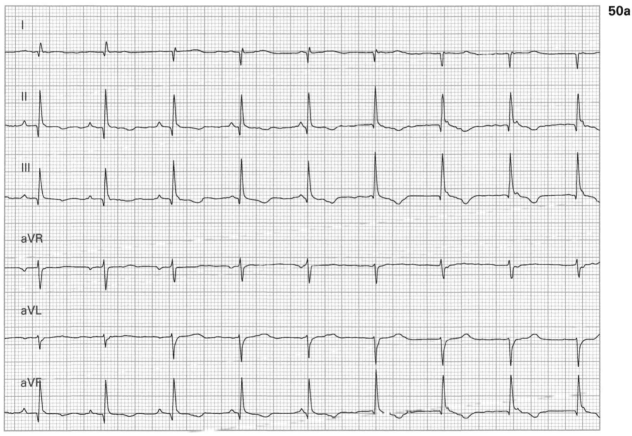

50a

Answer 50

1 The ventricular rate is 150 bpm. The P waves do not appear to be related to the QRS complexes. At the beginning of the recording the P waves (arrows) are in front of the QRS complexes but "drift" closer to, and then into and past, the QRS complexes in the middle and end of the recording (**ECG 50b**). Thus, there is no relationship between the P wave and QRS complexes indicating that two different independent pacemakers are driving the atria and ventricles. In the case of the atria, it is most likely that the sinus node is controlling the atrial rate whereas the normal QRS morphology suggests that a pacemaker located in or near the AV nodal junction is controlling the ventricles at a rate similar to the sinus node. The ECG is best described as isorhythmic atrioventricular dissociation.

2 Isorhythmic atrioventricular dissociation is typically benign as the junctional rate approximates the normal sinus rate. Treatment of isorhythmic AV dissociation is typically not required. In the authors' experience, the rhythm most commonly occurs in cats and is seen during anesthesia, in cases of systemic disease, and, occasionally, in cases of underlying heart disease.

50b

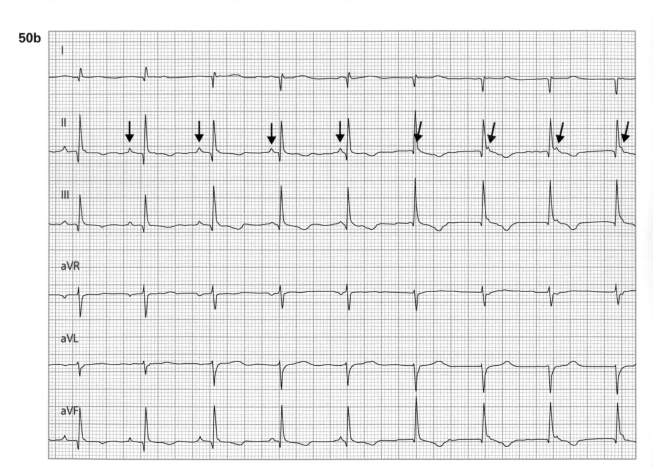

Question 51

ECG recorded from an ambulatory ECG (Holter) monitor in a dog.

1 What are the findings in **ECG 51a** (25 mm/sec; 10 mm/mV)?
2 What is the clinical significance of the ECG?

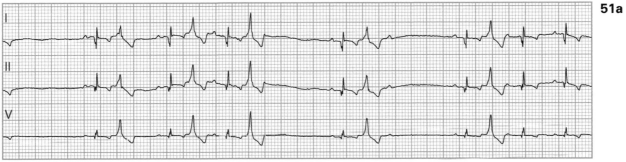

51a

Answer 51

1 The heart rate is irregular with an average rate of approximately 115 bpm. There appears to be occasional normal sinus beats (blue arrows) and frequent single ventricular premature beats (blue arrowheads) (**ECG 51b**). The PR interval of the third and sixth sinus beats (green bar), which immediately follow a VPC, appear prolonged at 0.16 second and 0.17 second, respectively. After the fourth VPC, there is a P wave (green arrowhead) without a QRS complex, indicating AV nodal block. The ECG findings are most consistent with sinus rhythm with single VPCs and concealed AV nodal conduction. Concealed AV nodal conduction refers to the assumption that the VPC was able to retrograde conduct into the AV node and partially or fully depolarize the AV nodal tissue, which resulted either in slow AV nodal conduction of the subsequent sinus beat (first-degree AV nodal block) or intermittent failure of the sinus impulses to traverse the AV node and cause a subsequent QRS complex (second-degree AV nodal block). The term "concealed" refers to the fact that the depolarization of the AV node is not actually detected on the ECG, only the effect that it has on subsequent sinus beats.

2 Concealed AV nodal conduction is relatively common in the presence of VPCs and contributes to the pauses following VPCs. No specific treatment is needed to address concealed conduction and the occasional dropped P wave. The VPCs can be due to underlying heart disease, such as cardiomyopathy or valvular disease or secondary to extracardiac causes such as abdominal disease or other systemic conditions.

51b

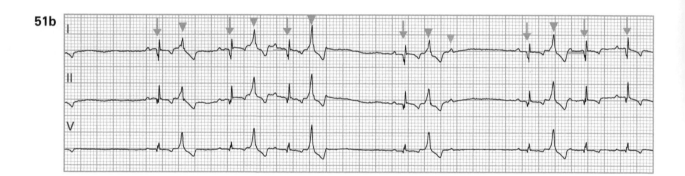

NEW ADVANCED-LEVEL ECG CASES

Question 52
ECG recorded from a dog with a history of weakness and tachycardia.

1 What are the findings in **ECG 52** (50 mm/sec; 10 mm/mV)?
2 What is the clinical significance of this ECG?

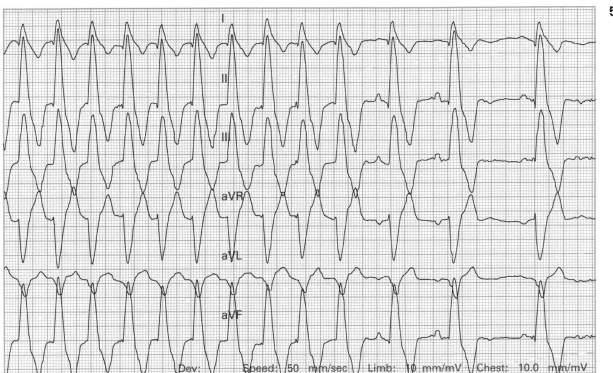

Answer 52

1 The heart rate at the beginning of the recording is 250 bpm and at the end of the recording is 110 bpm. The first part of the recording is best described as a "wide complex" tachycardia, which could be due to ventricular tachycardia or supraventricular tachycardia with a concurrent conduction abnormality, such as a left bundle branch block. In the second half of the recording, the tachycardia is disrupted, resulting in a marked decrease in heart rate and P waves are visible preceding each QRS complex, indicating the sinus node to be the origin of these beats. The QRS complexes of the sinus beats appear identical to the QRS complexes during the supraventricular tachycardia and are abnormally wide (0.10 second), consistent with a left bundle branch block. Thus, the most likely ECG diagnosis is supraventricular tachycardia with a left bundle branch block. This type of wide complex supraventricular tachycardia is difficult to distinguish from ventricular tachycardia up until the point when the tachycardia is disrupted and P waves become apparent.

2 Left bundle branch block is usually associated with clinically important heart disease. Supraventricular tachycardia is often the result of underlying heart disease, especially diseases that are typified by atrial enlargement, such as mitral valve disease or dilated cardiomyopathy. Vagal maneuvers such as ocular pressure can be used to acutely disrupt supraventricular tachycardia and help distinguish supraventricular vs. ventricular tachycardia. Weakness, activity intolerance, or syncope can occur secondary to the tachycardia, especially if underlying myocardial disease is present. Treatment might include drugs that slow AV nodal conduction, such as diltiazem or atenolol, to reduce the ventricular heart rate.

Question 53

ECG recorded from a dog with tachycardia.

1 What are the findings in **ECG 53** (25 mm/sec; 20 mm/mV)?
2 What is the clinical significance of this ECG?

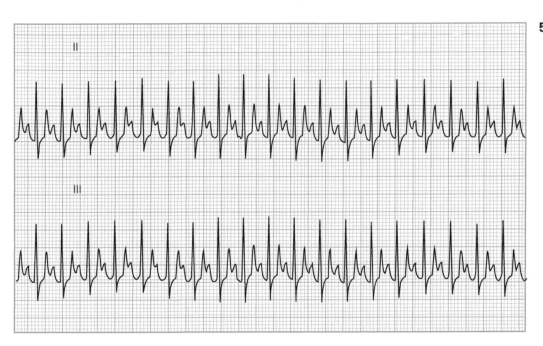

53

Answer 53

1 The heart rate is 215 bpm. The QRS complexes are narrow and appear to be of supraventricular origin, and there is a P wave with a consistent PR interval in front of each QRS complex. The most likely ECG diagnosis is supraventricular tachycardia.

2 Supraventricular tachycardia can arise secondary to underlying heart disease, especially diseases that are associated with atrial enlargement such as dilated cardiomyopathy or mitral valve disease. Dogs can exhibit signs of weakness, lethargy, exercise intolerance, or syncope due to the rapid heart rate. Treatment might involve vagal maneuver to acutely slow or disrupt the tachycardia and parenteral or oral drugs, such as diltiazem or beta-blockers, to slow AV nodal conduction.

Question 54
ECG recorded from a young dog with tachycardia and episodic weakness.

1 What are the findings in **ECG 54a** (50 mm/sec; 10 mm/mV)?
2 What is the clinical significance of this ECG?

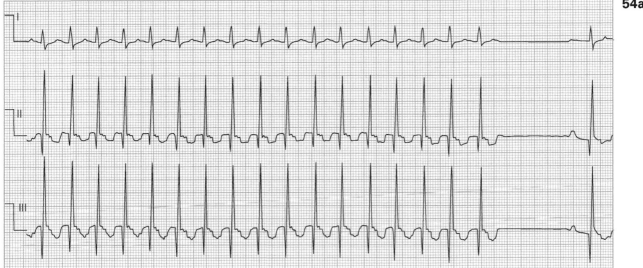

54a

Answer 54

1 The heart rate during the majority of the recording is 275 bpm. The QRS complex is narrow and positive in lead II and appears to be of supraventricular origin. Thus, supraventricular tachycardia is the most likely ECG diagnosis. There are small negative deflections in the ST segment of each QRS complex that are likely a retrograde P wave (P', arrows) and best seen in leads II and III. Toward the end of the recording, the supraventricular tachycardia is suddenly terminated and a normal sinus beat occurs after a pause (see Box). The presence of the P' wave and its close proximity to the preceding QRS complex is highly suggestive of a re-entrant mechanism due to an accessory pathway between the atrium and ventricle. These types of supraventricular arrhythmias are most commonly detected in Labrador Retrievers and are the result of an abnormal band of conduction tissue that provides a second connection between the atrium and ventricle in addition to the AV node (see boxed text below).

2 The rapid heart rate during supraventricular tachycardia can cause weakness, exercise intolerance, and syncope. Treatment consists of blocking the re-entrant circuit at the AV node using calcium channel blockers, beta-blocker, or digoxin, and at the accessory pathway using sodium-channel or potassium-channel blockers. Catheter-based radiofrequency ablation of the accessory pathway can also be performed but is limited to a small number of centers worldwide.

Re-entrant supraventricular tachycardia due to accessory pathways

(A) Accessory pathways involve conduction tissue between the atrium and ventricle independent of the AV node. During the most common type of supraventricular tachycardia associated with accessory pathways, an impulse travels from the atrium across the AV node and into the ventricle (1), resulting in a normal appearing QRS complex (2). The ventricular action potential is then able to conduct from the ventricle back into the atrium, using the accessory pathway, which depolarizes the atrium in a retrograde fashion and produces a retrograde (i.e., negative) P wave within the ST segment of the preceding QRS complex (3). The impulse then re-enters the AV node (4) and the cycle repeats itself producing a supraventricular tachycardia (B). The re-entry circuit involves both the AV node and the accessory pathway, and these two areas represent potential targets to disrupt and terminate the tachycardia using antiarrhythmic drugs or catheter-based radiofrequency ablation.

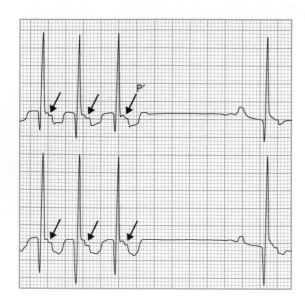

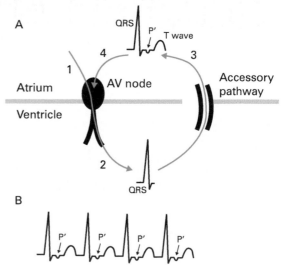

Question 55

ECG recorded in a 12-year-old Saluki diagnosed with fainting due to third-degree AV nodal block. A single-chamber pacemaker was implanted, which alleviated clinical signs. The patient presents 8 months later for collapsing.

1 What are the findings in **ECG 55a** (50 mm/sec; 5 mm/mV)?
2 What is the clinical significance of this ECG?
3 What further diagnostics should be considered?

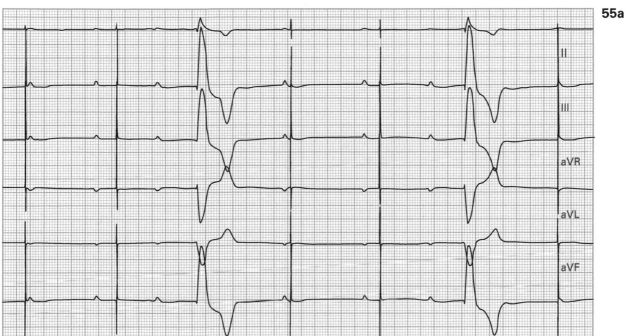

55a

Answer 55

1 **ECG 55a** shows failure of the pacemaker to capture. The underlying rhythm is third-degree AV nodal block. Ventricular pacing spikes (blue arrows) represent the electrical output from the pacemaker and can be seen occurring at regular intervals (every 0.67 second) but without any pacing-induced QRS complexes following each spike (**ECG 55b**). Because of the failure of the pacemaker to control heart rate in the presence of the AV nodal block, ventricular escape beats have appeared (black arrows).

2 This patient collapsed because there were long periods of asystole occurring due to the loss of capture from the malfunctioning pacemaker.

3 A chest radiograph and a pacemaker interrogation should be performed. The chest radiograph will allow to see if the pacemaker lead is displaced or in its original position. The pacemaker interrogation assesses electrical parameters such as output voltage and duration. Common causes of loss of capture include lead dislodgement, insufficient pacing voltage or duration, or lead fracture. In this patient, radiographs confirmed that the pacemaker lead was in place. The output voltage was increased, which resulted in successful and consistent capture of the ventricle and creating a pacing-induced QRS complex.

55b

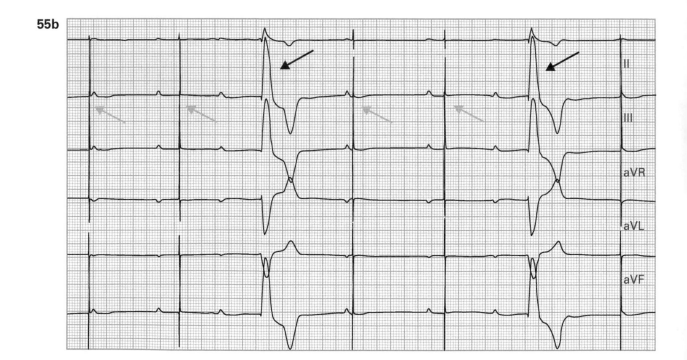

Question 56

ECG recorded in a 8-year-old West Highland White Terrier collapsing because of sick sinus syndrome. A pacemaker was implanted without complications and set to pace at 110 bpm.

1 What are the findings in **ECG 56a** (50 mm/sec; 10 mm/mV)?
2 What re-programming can be done to resolve the problem?

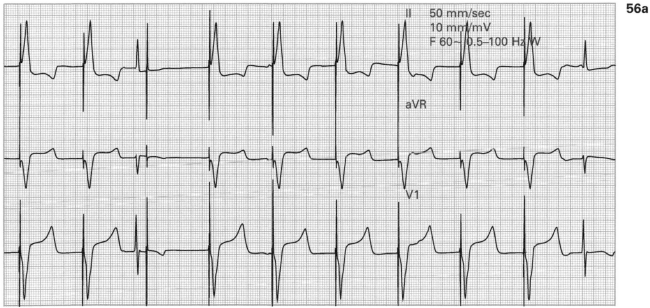

56a

II 50 mm/sec
10 mm/mV
F 60~ 0.5–100 Hz W

aVR

V1

Answer 56

1　**ECG 56a** shows that the pacemaker is undersensing the dog's intrinsically generated (native) QRS complexes. This occurs when the pacemaker does not sense or detect the intrinsic QRS complex (black arrow) and continues to pace and deliver an electrical output (i.e., pacing spike) (blue arrow) when it should be resting (**ECG 56b**). This pacing spike also demonstrates loss of capture; it does not cause a subsequent QRS complex because the pacemaker delivered the stimulus during the ST segment (i.e., ventricular refractory period) of the preceding intrinsic beat and could not stimulate a ventricular depolarization. This is a potentially dangerous scenario as delivery of pacing spike during this vulnerable period of repolarization can induce ventricular fibrillation (VF). The greens arrows represent a pacing spike followed by subsequent capture and a paced QRS complex.

2　Sensitivity refers to the minimum electrical voltage that the pacemaker will detect as a native depolarization. For example, a sensitivity of 3 mV means that the pacemaker will only sense a signal equal to or greater than 3 mV. The pacemaker ignores all other voltages. Thus, one cause of undersensing is that the sensitivity setting is higher than the voltage of the native QRS depolarizations at the pacemaker lead tip. To correct undersensing, the ventricular sensitivity of the pacemaker is increased by decreasing the threshold value. In this case, the sensing value was decreased to 2.5 mV. **ECG 56c** shows that the change in sensitivity resulted in the pacemaker appropriately sensing the intrinsic beats and only pacing when the intrinsic rate falls below 110 bpm.

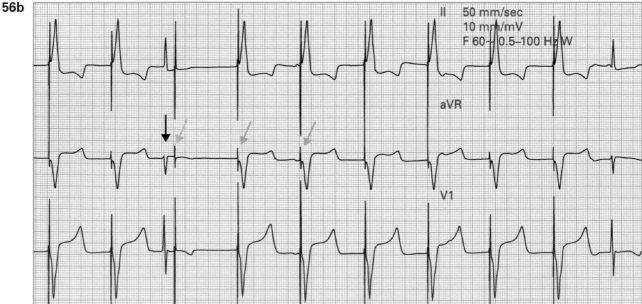

56b

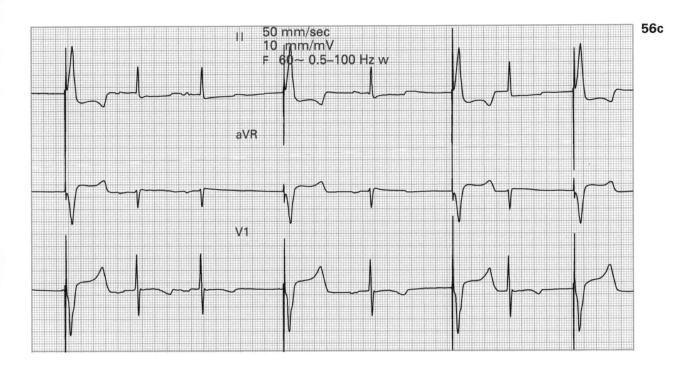

56c

Question 57

ECG recorded in a 13-year-old mixed breed dog that originally presented for collapsing due to complete AV nodal block. A pacemaker was implanted and set to pace at 75 bpm.

1 What are the findings in **ECG 57a** (25 mm/sec; 10 mm/mV)?
2 What re-programming can be done to resolve the problem?

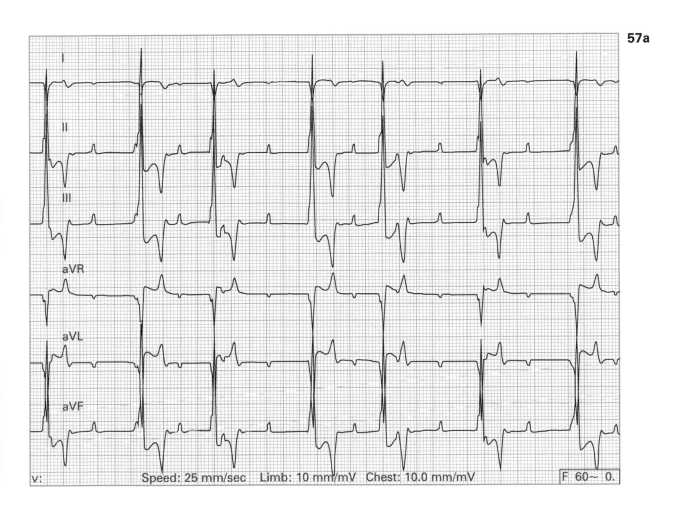

57a

Answer 57

1 ECG 57a shows that the pacemaker is oversensing. The pacemaker occasionally detects the T wave and mistakes it for an intrinsically generated QRS complex. The pacemaker is programmed to pace at 75 bpm (i.e., time between ventricular paced [VP] beats of 800 ms). In this example, the pacemaker senses the T wave (VS = ventricular sense, horizontal blue arrow) and waits to pace again 800 ms after the sensed T wave (**ECG 57b**). This results in a R-R interval that is longer than 800 ms (green arrow) and heart rate slower than 75 bpm each time the pacemaker senses the T waves.

2 Oversensing can result in pacing at a lower than expected rate as the inappropriate detection inhibits the pacemaker from pacing at the correct rate. As described in Question 56, sensitivity refers to the minimum electrical voltage that the pacemaker will detect as a native depolarization. Oversensing occurs if the pacemaker senses electric signals, such as skeletal muscle myopotentials, electromagnetic interference, or P or T waves and interprets them as native QRS complexes. The likelihood of oversensing can be increased by inadequate programming of sensitivity settings or refractory periods, lead or device failure, or changes in signal amplitude due to change in tissue characteristics that can occur over time (i.e., fibrosis. hyperkalemia). In most cases, the inappropriately sensed electrical events are of lower voltage than the true QRS complexes, and decreasing the pacemaker's ventricular sensitivity will correct the problem. In this case, the sensing threshold value was increased from 3.8 to 5.0 mV, and the oversensing was corrected.

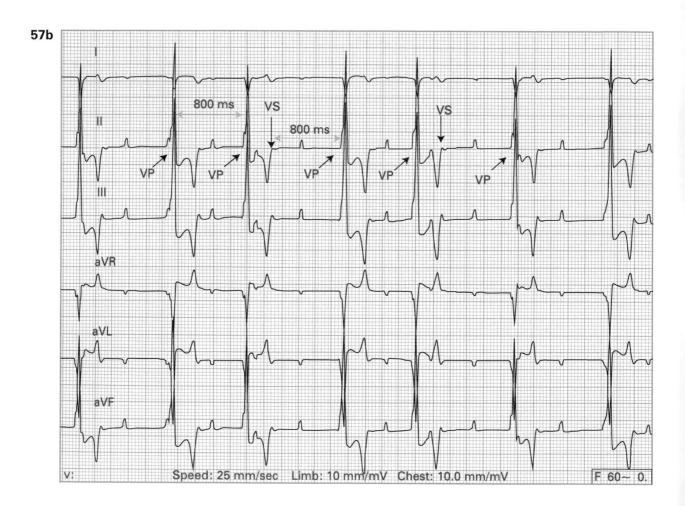

57b

NEW HOLTER MONITORING ECG CASES

Question 58

Holter recording summary from a 6-year-old male, castrated Boxer with a history of ventricular premature complexes (VPCs) and ventricular tachycardia (VT) on an in-hospital ECG, due to arrhythmogenic right ventricular cardiomyopathy (ARVC). The summary displays the number of VPCs and runs of VT during the 24-hour recording period as well as the VPCs as a percentage of the total QRS complexes. Antiarrhythmic therapy was started (sotalol 2 mg/kg q 12 h PO) to suppress the ventricular arrhythmias. A recheck Holter recording was acquired after 1 week of sotalol therapy.

	VPCs/24 h	Runs of VT/24 h	Ventricular ectopic beats as percentage of total number of beats/24 h
Pre-treatment	5,822	42	6.2%
Sotalol	14,681	295	13.8%

1 What is the interpretation of the Holter recording results?
2 What recommendations regarding drug therapy might be made?

Answer 58

1 The arrhythmia count has markedly increased under sotalol therapy, indicating a proarrhythmic effect by this potassium-channel blocking agent in this dog.
2 The goal is to reduce the number of VPCs by >80% in order to account for day-to-day variation in the number of VPCs. Sotalol failed to decrease the total number of VPCs. An antiarrhythmic with a different mechanism of action might be tried. In this case, sotalol was replaced with mexiletine (sodium-channel blocker) and atenolol (beta-blocker) and eliminated of runs of VT and reduced total ventricular ectopy percentage to <0.1%.

Treatment	VPC/24 h	Runs of VT/24 h	Ventricular ectopic beats as percentage of total number of beats/24 h
Pre-treatment	5,822	42	6.2%
Sotalol	14,681	295	13.8%
Mexiletine *plus* atenolol	29	0	<0.1%

Question 59

Holter recording summary from a 4-year-old female, spayed Boxer that fainted while jogging with the owner and had runs of ventricular tachycardia (VT) on an in-hospital ECG. Treatment with sotalol at 1.5 mg/kg q 12 h was initiated. One week later, a Holter recording was acquired. (VPCs, ventricular premature contractions.)

Time	Treatment	VPC/24 h	Runs of VT/24 h	Ventricular ectopic beats as percentage of total number of beats/24 h
+1 week	Sotalol 1.5 mg/kg BID	6,415	33	6.2%

1 What is your interpretation of the Holter recording results?
2 What recommendations regarding drug therapy might be made?
3 What recommendations regarding arrhythmia monitoring might be made?

Answer 59

1 The clinical signs at presentation suggested a high risk of sudden death and prompted the start of antiarrhythmic therapy. Thus, Holter data prior to start of sotalol are not available for comparison and whether or not sotalol reduced the baseline number of VPCs is uncertain; however, the total number of VPCs while receiving sotalol is relatively high.

2 The initial dose of sotalol is at the lower end of the dose range (1.5–2.5 mg/kg q 12 h), and the dose was increased to 2.2 mg/kg q 12 h. A repeat Holter 1 week later revealed a decrease in number of VPCs of >98% as compared with the previous recording.

Time	Treatment	VPC/24 h	Runs of VT/24 h	Ventricular ectopic beats as percentage of total number of beats/24 h
+1 week	Sotalol 1.5 mg/kg BID	6,415	33	6.2%
+2 weeks	Sotalol 2.2 mg/kg BID	84	0	<0.1%

3 Control of arrhythmias can change over time as the underlying disease progresses. Repeat Holter recordings at 6–12-month intervals are often considered, depending on the severity and complexity of the initial arrhythmias or recurrence of clinical signs. Consider the follow-up Holter results obtained 6 months later, which showed apparent loss of efficacy of the sotalol.

Time	Treatment	VPC/24 h	Runs of VT/24 h	Ventricular ectopic beats as percentage of total number of beats/24 h
+6 months	Sotalol 2.2 mg/kg BID	23,102	425	21.0%

Inadequate arrhythmic suppression with sotalol might benefit from the addition of mexiletine and, in this case, resulted in marked reduction of VPCs, although there were still 18 runs of VT.

Time	Treatment	VPC/24 h	Runs of VT/24 h	Ventricular ectopic beats as percentage of total number of beats/24 h
+7 months	Sotalol 2.2 mg/kg BID *plus* Mexiletine 5.5 mg/kg	302	18	<1.0%

Question 60

Holter recording summary from a Doberman Pinscher with a history of advanced dilated cardiomyopathy, recent recurrence of congestive heart failure and a rapid irregular rhythm. An ECG recording revealed atrial fibrillation with a heart rate >250 bpm. Treatment with diltiazem and digoxin was initiated. A 24-hour Holter recording was obtained 1 week later. At that visit, the congestive heart failure was well controlled, but the dog was reported to have lost his appetite over the last 2 days. (VPCs, ventricular premature contractions; VT, ventricular tachycardia.)

Time	Treatment	24 h mean HR	VPC/24 h	Runs of VT/24 h	Ventricular ectopic beats as percentage of total number of beats/24 h
+1 week	Diltiazem XR: 3.8 mg/kg BID Digoxin: 0.004 mg/kg BID	167	17,903	2	7.6%

1 What is your interpretation of the Holter recording results?
2 What recommendations regarding drug therapy might be made?

Answer 60

1 The 2-hour mean HR is 167 bpm, which is elevated and indicates poor control of the ventricular rate secondary to atrial fibrillation. There are frequent VPCs and two runs of VT, which suggest a high risk for sudden death. The goal is to reduce the 24-hour mean heart rate to 125 bpm or lower.

2 Inappetence is a common side effect of digoxin in dogs. Serum digoxin levels at 6–8 hours post-pill are routinely performed 1 week after starting the treatment. Dobermans are particularly sensitive and can experience gastrointestinal side effects even at low serum levels. Digoxin can also induce ventricular arrhythmias, and for these reasons, digoxin was discontinued. Diltiazem, while useful for atrial fibrillation, does not suppress ventricular arrhythmias and an additional antiarrhythmic was prescribed. Because of the poor contractility associated with advanced DCM in this case, sotalol was not used. Instead, amiodarone therapy was initiated (10 mg/kg BID for 1-week loading dose followed by maintenance dose of 6.5 mg/kg BID), and a repeat Holter recording was acquired 4 weeks later. The 24 h mean HR was reduced (albeit still above the desired 125 bpm) and the ventricular ectopy and VT was deemed adequately controlled. (See also Chapter 5, Fig. 5.8.)

Time	Treatment	24 h mean HR	VPC/24 h	Runs of VT/24 h	Total ventricular percentage ectopy
+1 week	Diltiazem XR: 3.8 mg/kg BID Digoxin: 0.004 mg/kg BID	167	17,903	2	7.6%
+4 weeks	Diltiazem XR: 3.8 mg/kg BID Amiodarone: 6.5 mg/kg BID	138	1,901	0	1.0%

Question 61

ECGs recorded from a dog under anesthesia

1 What are the findings in **ECGs 61a** and **61b** (25 mm/sec; 10 mm/mV)?

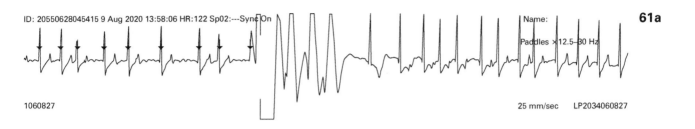

61a

ID: 20550628045415 9 Aug 2020 13:58:06 HR:122 Sp02:---Sync On

Name:

Paddles x 12.5–30 Hz

1060827

25 mm/sec   LP2034060827

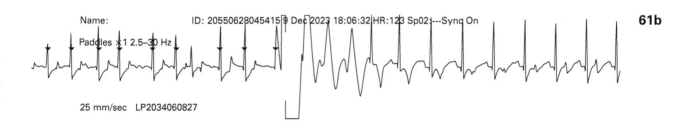

61b

Name:

Paddles x 1 2.5–30 Hz

ID: 20550628045415 9 Dec 2023 18:06:32 HR:123 Sp02:---Sync On

25 mm/sec   LP2034060827

Answer 61

1 ECGs **61a** and **61b** demonstrate two separate attempts at electrical cardioversion of atrial fibrillation.
- The beginning of each of the traces shows an irregular rhythm with a narrow (i.e., supraventricular) QRS complex. Distinct P waves are not visible, but rather an undulating baseline representative of F waves. Findings are consistent with atrial fibrillation.
- The arrowheads at the beginning of each of the tracings demonstrate appropriate "syncing" by the cardioversion unit with the QRS complexes. A large, biphasic deflection represents the shock delivery (blue arrow), which is synchronized with a QRS complex. The defibrillation attempt was performed using a biphasic shock.
- **ECG 61a** was recorded during a shock of 2 J/kg. The shock is followed by three beats of a wide complex tachycardia that likely is ventricular tachycardia, before resumption of atrial fibrillation. Failure of successful conversion can be due to failure to depolarize >75% of the atrial myocardium or if the cardioversion paddles are not in an optimal position on the dog's chest. In these instances, the cardioversion energy can be increased, the paddles can be repositioned, or both.
- **ECG 61b** demonstrates a subsequent and successful electrical conversion of atrial fibrillation of the dog in **ECG 61a**. The beginning of the trace shows atrial fibrillation with synchronization markers similar to **ECG 61a**, however, the seventh QRS complex is not appropriately identified by the defibrillator and is missing a QRS marker. The energy required for cardioversion using a biphasic defibrillator ranges between 0.5–3 J/kg. A shock of 3 J/kg (blue arrow) was delivered directly after a QRS complex. A short run of ventricular tachycardia is then followed by a regular supraventricular rhythm with distinct P waves (green arrows) and is most consistent with sinus rhythm. Cardioversion commonly induces brief ventricular arrhythmias or pauses before atrial fibrillation returns or sinus rhythm resumes. In this case, an increase in cardioversion energy from 2 to 3 J/kg resulted in successful termination of atrial fibrillation and sinus rhythm was restored.

61a

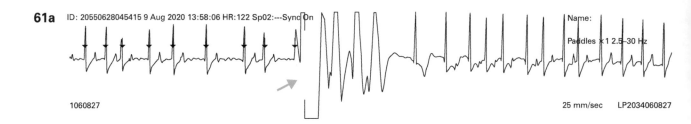

ID: 205506280454415 9 Aug 2020 13:58:06 HR:122 Sp02:---Sync On

Name:

Paddles x1 2.5–30 Hz

1060827

25 mm/sec   LP2034060827

61b

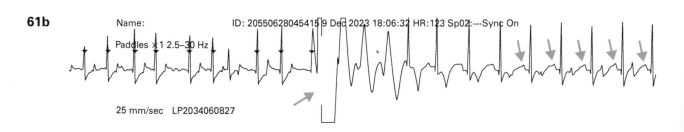

Name:

Paddles x1 2.5–30 Hz

ID: 205506280454415 9 Dec 2023 18:06:32 HR:123 Sp02:---Sync On

25 mm/sec   LP2034060827

Electrical cardioversion of atrial fibrillation has similarities to electrical defibrillation of ventricular fibrillation (see Case 25). Similar to ventricular defibrillation, cardioversion of atrial fibrillation is accomplished by delivering an electrical shock to the heart, thereby depolarizing the majority of the cardiac muscle. The myocardium becomes temporarily inexcitable, causing disruption of the arrhythmia reentry circuits and promoting the return of sinus rhythm. Unlike ventricular defibrillation, cardioversion of atrial fibrillation is specifically timed with the QRS complex so as to avoid shock delivery during the T wave and the relative refractory portion of the cardiac cycle, which can induce ventricular fibrillation.

Defibrillators suitable for cardioversion of atrial fibrillation have capability to be set to a SYNC mode so the synchronizing circuit within the defibrillator will detect the patient's R or S waves. Newer defibrillation units deliver biphasic shocks, which are effective at lower energy levels as compared with monophasic shocks. During cardioversion of atrial fibrillation, the SHOCK button is pressed and held, and the unit automatically discharges during the next detected R or S wave. When in SYNC mode, the unit displays arrow markers that the operator can examine to ensure accurate identification of QRS complex. For a biphasic defibrillator, the recommended initial shock energy for an external cardioversion of atrial fibrillation using paddles or patches is 0.5–3 J/kg body weight. If the first shock is not effective, additional single shocks of increasing energy are delivered. Shock delivery is extremely painful and the patient with atrial fibrillation has to be anesthetized. The dog is placed in dorsal or lateral recumbency and self-adhesive defibrillation pads or handheld defibrillation paddles are applied on opposites sides of the chest following application of conductive paste or gel.

REFERENCE GUIDE

PAPER SPEED AND SENSITIVITY

Paper speed	Each 1 mm along x-axis
25 mm/sec	0.04 sec
50 mm/sec	0.02 sec

Sensitivity	Each 1 mm along y-axis
10 mm/mV	0.1 mV

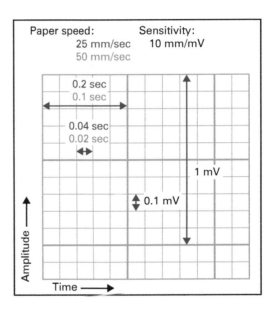

Paper speed: 25 mm/sec / 50 mm/sec   Sensitivity: 10 mm/mV

0.2 sec / 0.1 sec

0.04 sec / 0.02 sec

1 mV

0.1 mV

Amplitude

Time

NORMAL ECG AMPLITUDES AND DURATIONS IN THE DOG AND CAT

	Dog	Cat
Heart rate	Puppy: 70–220 bpm Adult: 70–180 bpm	120–240 bpm
Rhythm	Sinus rhythm Sinus arrhythmia	Sinus rhythm
P wave		
Amplitude	Max: 0.4 mV	Max: 0.2 mV
Duration	Max: 0.04 s	Max: 0.04 s
PR interval	0.06–0.13 s	0.05–0.09 s
QRS		
Amplitude	Max: 2.5 mV, small breeds (3.0 mV, large breeds)	Max: 0.9 mV
Duration	0.06 s	0.04 s
ST segment	Not elevated or depressed >0.2 mV	No elevation or depression
T wave	Positive, negative, or biphasic, not >25% height of R wave	Isoelectric or usually positive <0.3 mV
Electrical axis	+40° to +100°	0 to +160°

Source: Adapted from Tilley LP and Smith WK. In: Tilley LP et al., eds. *Manual of Canine and Feline Cardiology*, 4th ed. Saunders Elsevier, St. Louis: 2008.

ECG WAVEFORM AMPLITUDES AND DURATIONS

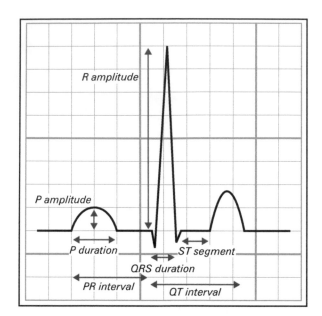

SIX-LEAD ECG AXIS SYSTEM

Mean electrical axis
Dog: +40° to +100°
Cat: 0° to +160°

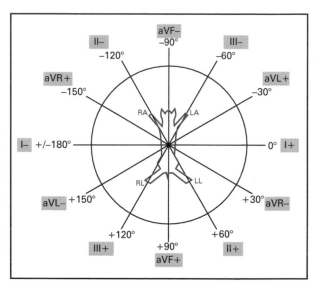

SELECTED ANTIARRHYTHMIC DRUGS

Drug	Dose	Indication
Lidocaine	*Dog:* 2 mg/kg IV bolus up to 3 times 30–80 μg/kg/min CRI	Ventricular tachycardia
Procainamide	*Dog:* 5–15 mg/kg IV bolus, slowly over 2 minutes 25–50 μg/kg/min CRI *Cat:* 2–5 μg/kg/min	Ventricular or supraventricular tachycardia
Sotalol	*Dog:* 1.0–2.0 mg/kg PO BID *Cat:* 10 mg/cat PO BID	Ventricular or supraventricular tachycardia
Atenolol	*Dog:* 0.25–2.0 mg/kg PO S-BID *Cat:* 6.25–12.5 mg/cat PO S-BID	Ventricular or supraventricular tachycardia
Diltiazem XR	*Dog:* 3–4 mg/kg PO BID *Cat:* 30–60 mg/cat PO S-BID	Atrial fibrillation or supraventricular tachycardia
Diltiazem	*Dog:* 0.5–2.0 mg/kg PO TID 0.1–0.2 mg/kg IV 2–6 mcg/kg/min CRI *Cat:* 1.0–2.5 mg/kg PO TID	Atrial fibrillation or supraventricular tachycardia
Digoxin	*Dog:* 0.003–0.005 mg/kg PO BID *Cat:* 0.03125 mg/cat PO q48 hrs	Atrial fibrillation or supraventricular tachycardia
Atropine	*Dog/Cat:* 0.01–0.04 mg/kg IV/IM/SC	Bradycardia
Glycopyrrolate	*Dog/Cat:* 0.005–0.01 mg/kg IV/IM	Bradycardia
Propantheline	*Dog:* 0.25–0.5 mg/kg PO B-TID	Bradycardia
Theophylline	*Dog:* 10–20 mg/kg PO BID *Cat:* 15–25 mg/kg PO SID	Bradycardia
Terbutaline	*Dog:* 1.25–5.0 mg/dog PO B-TID	Bradycardia

INDEX

Index

Index

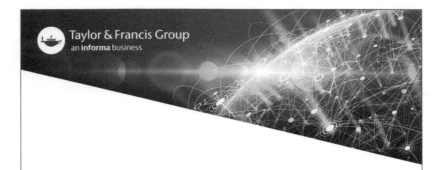

T - #0210 - 111024 - C156 - 261/194/7 - PB - 9780367146757 - Gloss Lamination